Frederick V. Nicolle M. CHIR., F.R.C.S

AESTHETIC RHINOPLASTY

W B Saunders Company Ltd
LONDON PHILADELPHIA TORONTO SYDNEY TOKYO

W. B. Saunders Company Ltd

24-28 Oval Road
London NW1 7DX

The Curtis Center
Independence Square West
Philadelphia, PA 19106-3399, USA

Harcourt Brace & Company
55 Horner Avenue
Toronto, Ontario M8Z 4X6, Canada

Harcourt Brace & Company, Australia
30-52 Smidmore Street
Marrickville, NSW 2204, Australia

Harcourt Brace & Company, Japan
Ichibancho Central Building, 22-1 Ichibancho
Chiyoda-ku, Tokyo 102, Japan

This book is printed on acid free paper

A catalogue record for this book is available from the British Library

ISBN 0-7020-1776-0

Typeset by Wordperfect Typesetters
Printed in Hong Kong by Dah Hua Printing Press Co Ltd

Contents

Contents

Part IV

Part V

Preface

Preface

The human nose denotes character of face and personality. It can depict sensuality or authority in its more flattering forms. It can also convey ugliness, meanness or the ridiculous in its other less flattering forms. It can also denote sex, changing age or ethnic origins.

Small wonder that such a feature as the nose has become an essential prop for the clown, or the pivotal feature of a drama such as Rostand's Cyrano de Bergerac. Could the quotation of Pascal 'Le nez de Cleopatre, s'il eût été plus court, toute la face de la terre aurait changé' suggest that even history has been influenced by an altered nose.?!

Lord Berners in his delightful book 'The Romance of a Nose', suggests that this really was so, and that Anthony's instant infatuation came about after Cleopatra's nose had been remodelled. Could this really be true? Investigation with the help of the British Museum shows an early bust of Cleopatra with a typical long Egyptian but unattractive heavy nose. Later the coinage minted with the head of Anthony and Cleopatra shows a much improved profile. We shall probably never know the truth although historically rhinoplasty was practised at such early times.

The demand for such surgical skills has continued and with this the quality of result has steadily improved. Technical skill has reached great levels but must always be sensitive and adaptable to the other human variables of character, sex, age and ethnic difference. This book aims to offer skills gained in the professional life of a plastic surgeon, as well as artistic perception, which add harmony and variation to the final results.

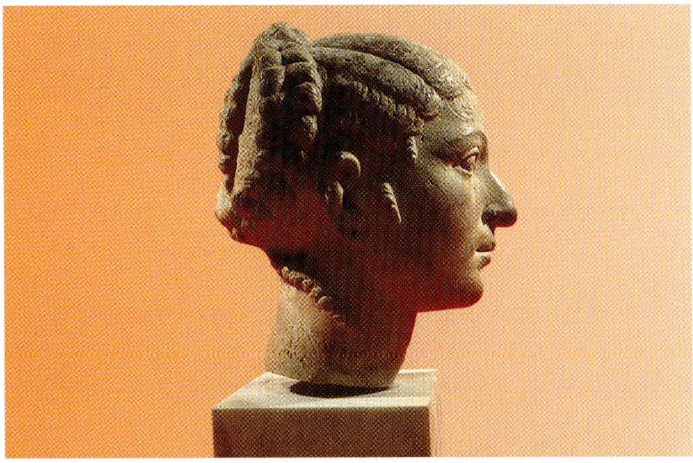

Bust of Cleopatara VII Queen of Egypt 51–30 BC (Roman Circa 30–40 BC).

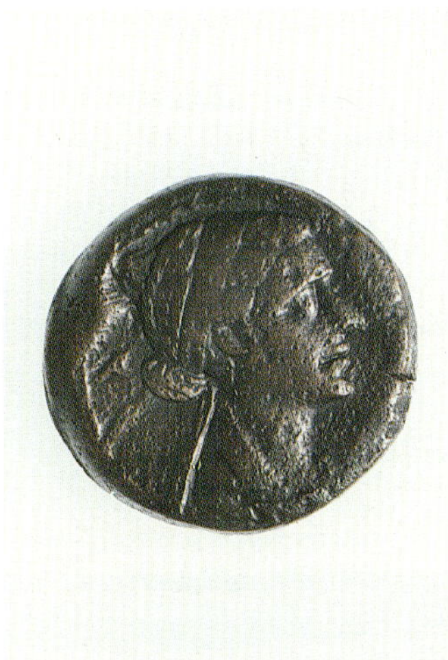

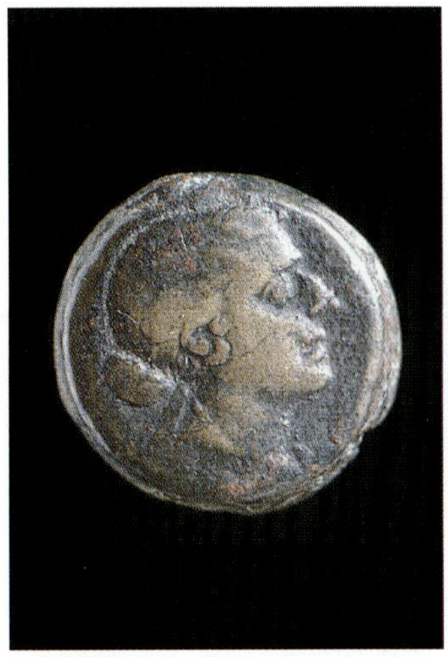

Coins showing heads of Anthony and Cleopatra.

Such a book required the skill of a particularly gifted illustrator, one who could appreciate and convey the importance of aesthetic as well as fine detail. I am greatly indebted to Anna Dutto for her co-operation and patience, and for her invaluable contribution.

This book would probably not have been completed if I had not had the inexhaustible help of my close colleague Basim Matti who devoted so many hours to assembling the illustrations from our extensive records, and has also given so much valuable and constructive criticism of the text.

I hope this book will stimulate as well as instruct those seeking the highest standards in one of the most demanding plastic surgical procedures.

References

The Romance of a Nose: by Lord Berners. Constable and Co: London, 1941.

Picture Credits

Part I

INTRODUCTION

Introduction

The nose commands such a dominant influence on facial appearance that it is not surprising that this subject has produced so many textbooks, and so many varying techniques.

Through my experience from my training, a clinical practice and teaching, for 10 years in North America and then for 20 years in England, I have been exposed to such diverse philosophies and techniques that it is evident that there is much for each continent to learn from the other. This experience has inevitably led to pressures and encouragement to produce my own textbook, which could be justified only if it offered new ideas and methods — not merely reproduction of material already covered in other excellent publications.

For this reason I have selected the patient approach and those techniques that I have found most valuable. Alternatives that I have not found to work as well in my own hands or those that appear in older textbooks but are not in common use have largely been excluded. Open rhinoplasty is not shown as I very seldom use it. In my opinion it should only be used for complex cases of septal deformity or cleft lip nose.

Rhinoplasty is an interplay between the nasal skeleton and the soft tissue skin cover. The interrelationship is best appreciated with the skin cover intact. Rhinoplasty is a highly skilled procedure and there no 'short cuts'.

The style of this book is similar to that of an illustrated lecture or what might be observed at operation. Throughout the pages the text is on the left with relevant illustrations on the right as far as possible. The photographic illustrations are of the highest possible standard in an attempt to maintain continuity of view point and scale, and for easy and accurate comparison. Newer techniques of colour illustration make a textbook of this quality possible at affordable prices and create a more stimulating and orderly presentation, approximating to live surgical demonstration.

Colour makes the details of surgical anatomy so much more easily recognizable. Where additional explanation is needed, the illustrations are supplemented with line drawings.

There is, however, an obvious danger for enthusiastic but inexperienced surgeons to concentrate on a technique before they have mastered the art of correct patient selection and assessment. This aspect is briefly considered first and references to more extensive texts offered. The ultimate surgical result will certainly require the highest technical skill, but without an aesthetic sense it will never achieve perfection. Aesthetic appreciation is therefore an essential ingredient which we must all strive to acquire and to apply, especially in those cases of subtle refinement, ethnic difference or differing age and sex.

Facial aesthetics and related anatomy

As with the assessment of a patient's psychological suitability, aesthetic appreciation comes naturally to some; it is a quality that can never fully be translated into lines and angles.

Basic understanding of facial proportions is best studied in any simple textbook about drawing of the human face and body; this is a most valuable exercise.

Descriptions in many surgical textbooks tend to encourage a point of view that is too stereotypical and it is better to see this subject through both an artist's and a surgeon's eye.

Once the basic skill of rhinoplasty is acquired we should strive to relate each nasal reconstruction not only to the individual's facial proportions but also to the age, sex and ethnic origins of the patient, and of course to the patient's expectations.

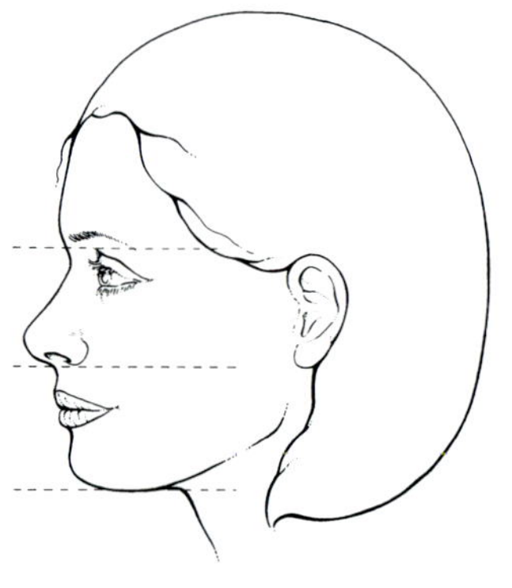

Figure 1.1

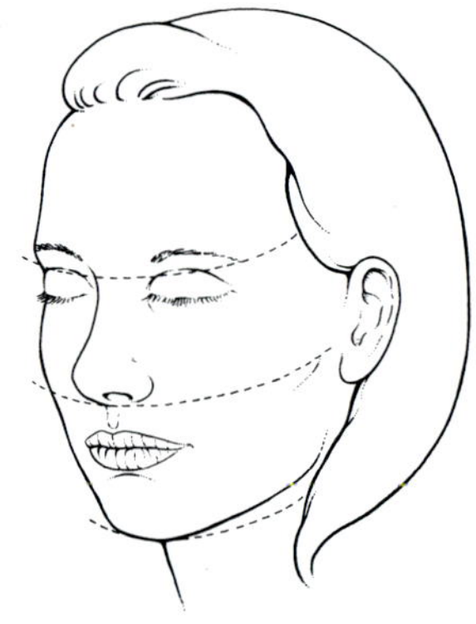

Figure 1.2

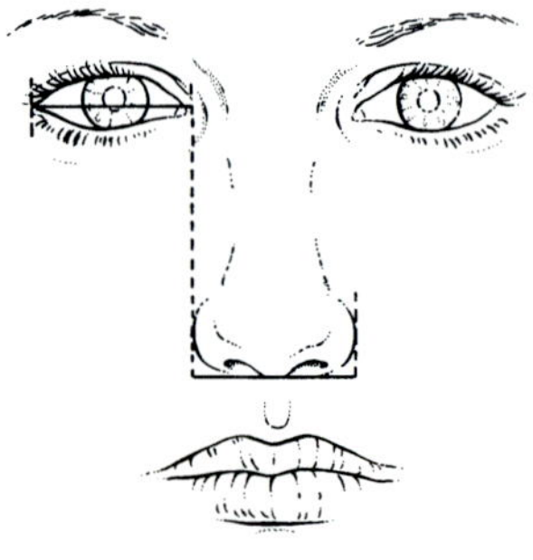

Figure 1.3

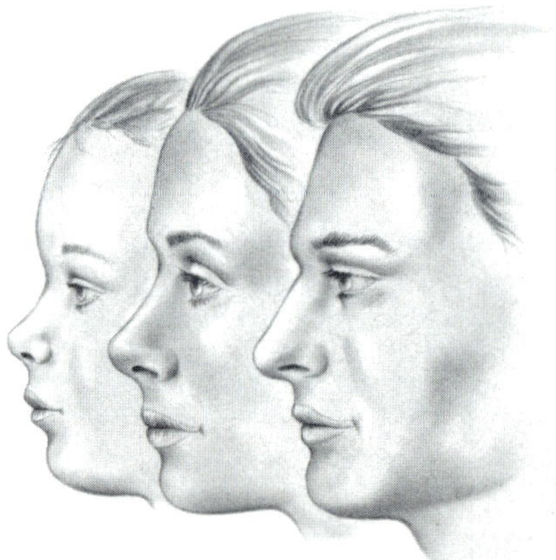

Figure 1.4

Nasal aesthetics

Variety

Much character is conveyed by the appearance of the nose and, for this reason, length as well as proportions are often exaggerated by the artist to convey greater effect.

In Europe, more than anywhere, the plastic surgeon is confronted with patients who display clear differences. In contrast, in North America both the USA and Canada have absorbed and cross-bred from a huge immigrant population during the last 300 years. Ethnic characteristics are given fuller consideration in Part V.

Surgeons must be more disciplined and accept what is real rather than ideal in their final objective.

The proportions of the nose vary with certain facial characteristics, thereby giving harmony, in spite of a wide variation in facial types.

For example:

- Negroid characteristics display wide lips and a wide nostril base.
- Aryan characteristics display finer lips and narrower nose.
- Jewish characteristics display pronounced cupids bow and a long nose with sharper angles.
- Latin characteristics display full lips and wider nasal tip.
- Oriental characteristics display softly defined lips and small child-like nose.

Basic harmony

Appreciation of the basic differences between rhinoplasty in the male and that in the female is discussed in the appropriate sections, but at this stage we need to train our eyes to recognize and then correct basic disproportion and disharmony.

Dorsum of the nose In the three-quarter view, the nose forms a smooth flowing curve from brow ridge to the nasal dorsum and tip. This line will vary, depending on the height of the radix and the width of the nasal bones.

In the lateral view the nose forms an angle with the vertical line of about 40° in males and 30° in females.

It is frequently stated that the tip should form the highest point on the dorsum. This may be true in the typically Oriental nose, but is likely to produce a child-like nose in other facial types. The most valid observation is that the tip should always lie higher than the supratip level. It is this that gives a pleasing form to both the aquiline Latin nose or that of any of the other European types.

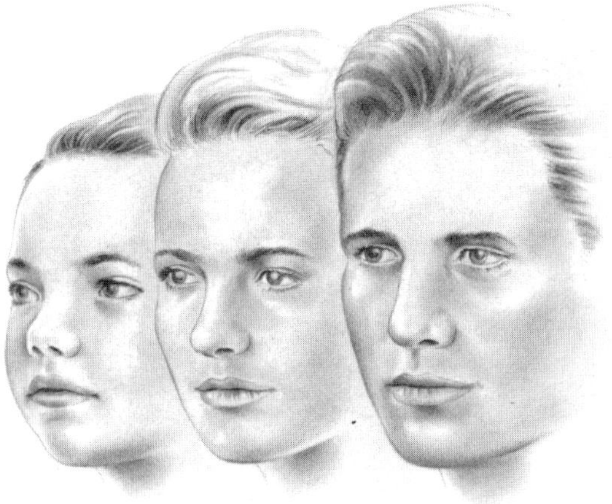

Figure 1.5

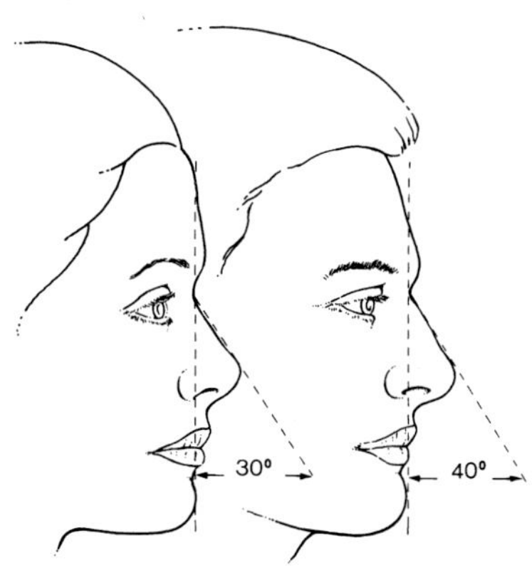

Figure 1.6

The tip of the nose This conveys sensitivity and should be angular rather than round. The lobular portion of the tip is triangular in outline and forms a diamond shape as it joins with the point of differentiation from the dorsum.

The nasocolumellar complex This is formed in a 2:1 ratio by the columella and the lobular portion of the tip, with a characteristic sharply defined angle at this junction.

The lip forms a soft angle with the inferior end of the columella making a wider angle in the female (110 – 115°) than in the male (90°).

The nostril margin forms a gentle concave curve running parallel with the columellar profile at a distance of 3 mm.

In noses of Oriental or Afro – Caribbean people this distance may be less and the concavity greater as a result of the more circular shape of the nostrils.

Much of the aesthetic harmony and subtle character of the nose is contained in this complex. Learn to develop the habit and skill of seeing through the skin, of recognizing the subtle features that are formed by the underlying variations in the tip cartilages to which the skin is tightly applied.

Basic variations

Apart from differing sexual and ethnic variations, the surgeon must recognize two forms of nose where very different techniques apply.

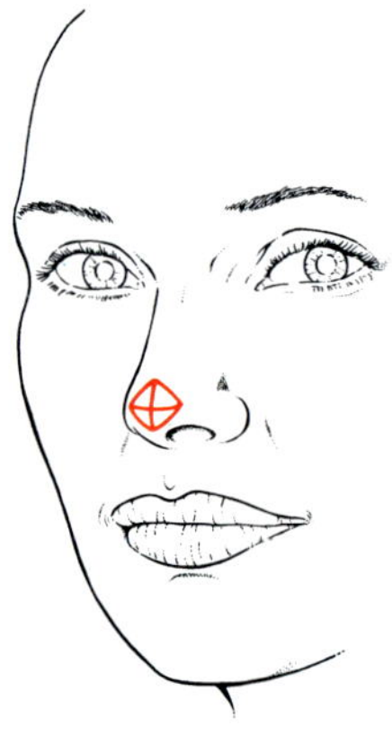

Figure 1.7a

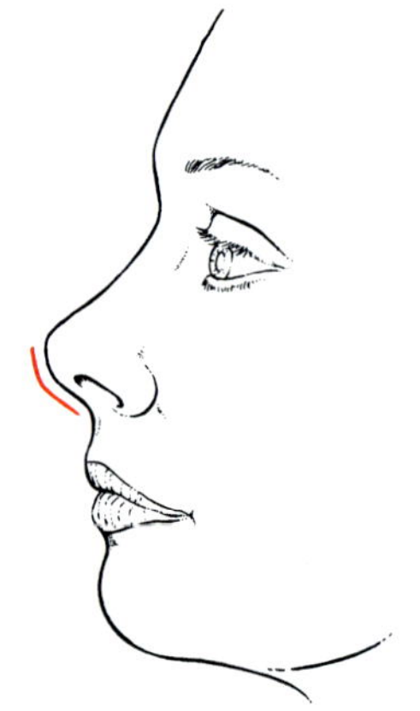

Figure 1.7b

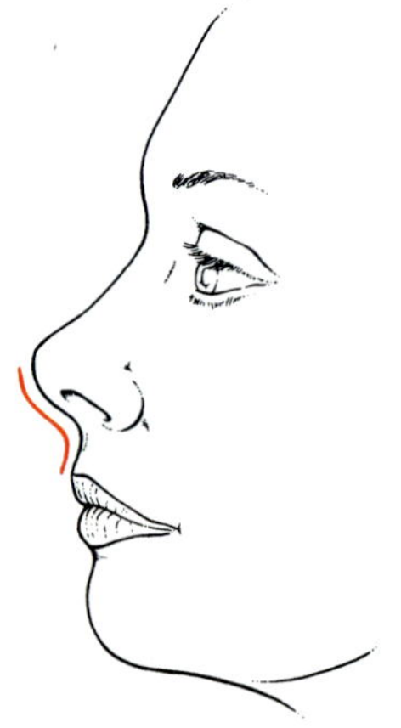

Figure 1.7c

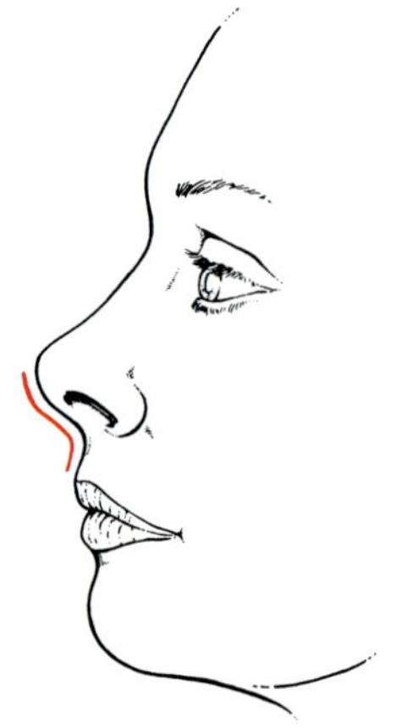

Figure 1.7d

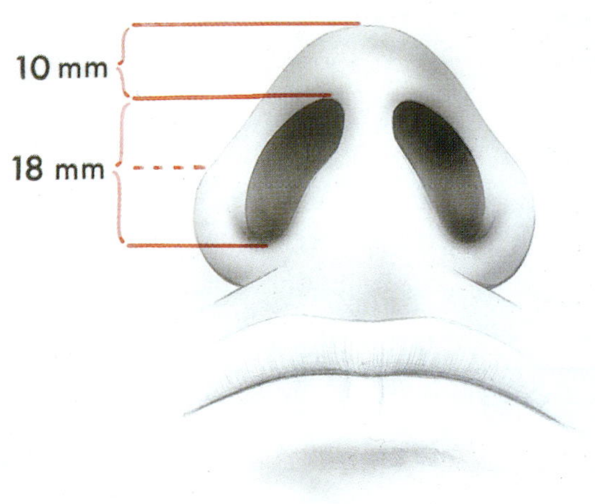

Figure 1.8

The 'top heavy' nose (Fig. 1.9) is usually characterized by a flat nasofrontal angle and high bony dorsum. Reduction of the bony component and high septum will result in aesthetic improvement.

The 'bottom heavy' nose (Fig. 1.10) has a low radix and relatively small nasal bones. The disproportion lies in the excessively large caudal components with large tip cartilages and variable excess of skin. Reduction is often extremely difficult and will need to be conservative. Overly ambitious reduction leads to inability of the skin cover to adapt to the reduced skeleton, with a resultant polly-beak deformity and hanging tip.

The surgeon learns to realize that some noses can be converted to a level of aesthetic perfection without a great deal of surgical contribution, whereas others demand the maximum surgical skills and yet are a minefield for the overconfident surgeon.

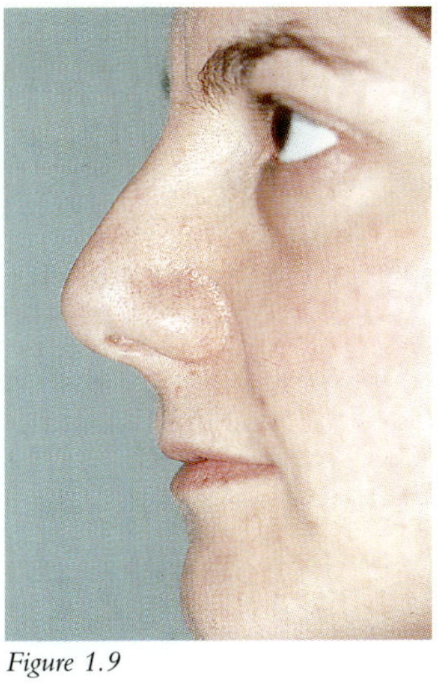

Figure 1.9

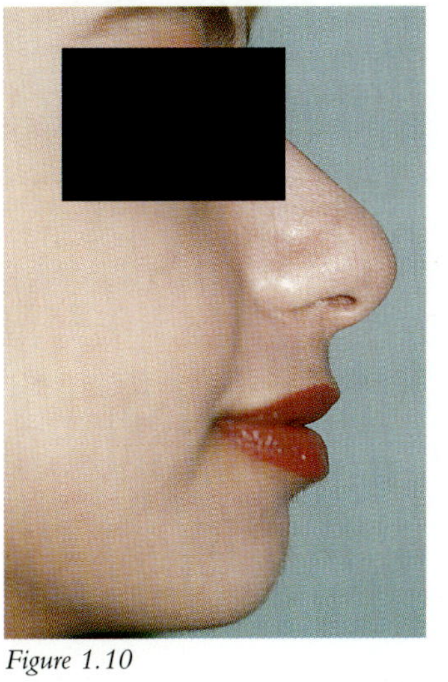

Figure 1.10

Figure 1.11 shows an example of a 'bottom heavy' nose with wide tip and wide nostril base. Conservative rhinoplasty, with narrowing of tip and reduction of alae procedures improved facial harmony and expression, as seen six months post-operatively.

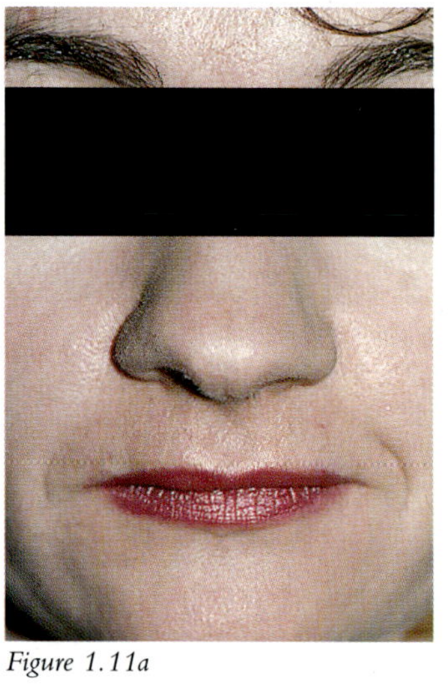

Figure 1.11a

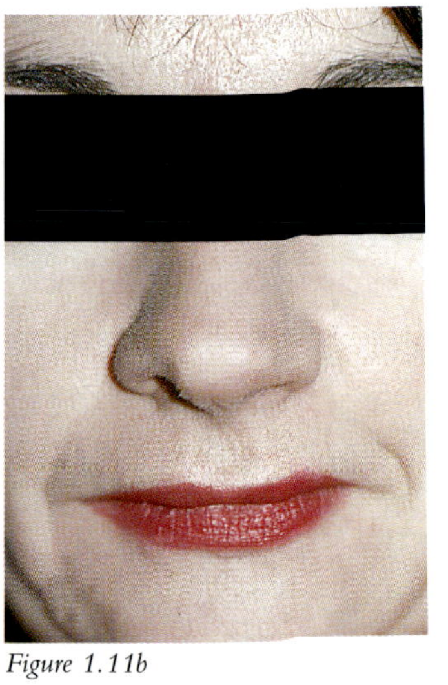

Figure 1.11b

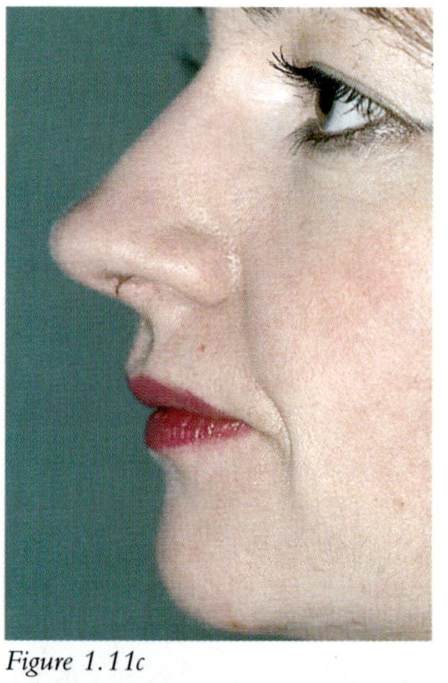

Figure 1.11c

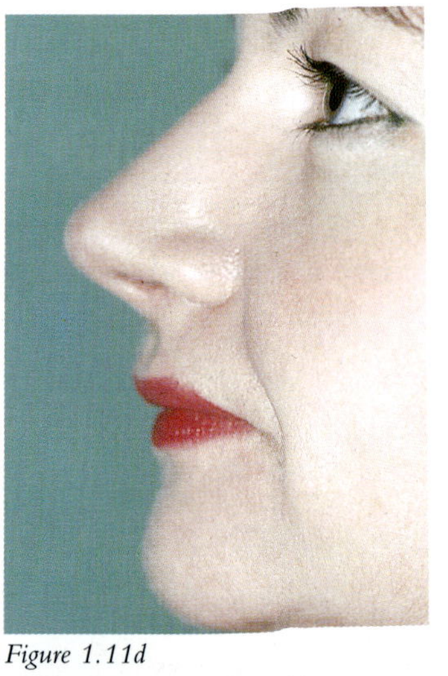

Figure 1.11d

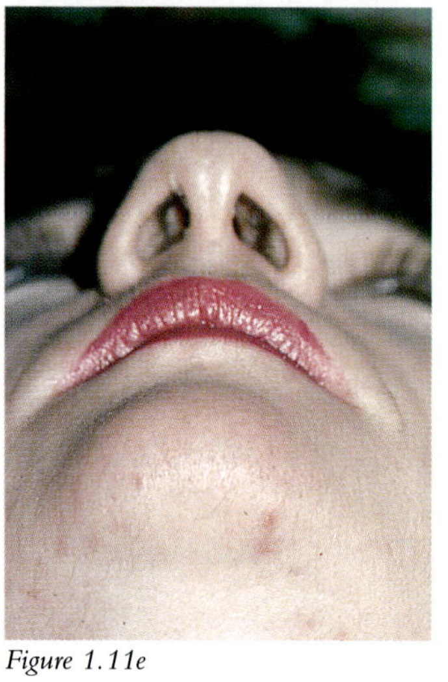

Figure 1.11e

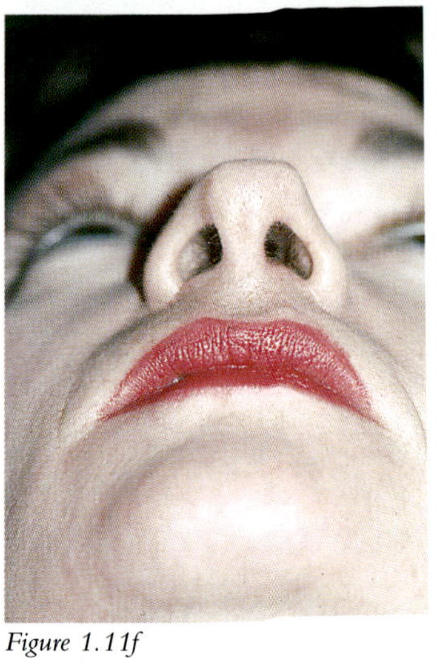

Figure 1.11f

Figure 1.12 shows an excellent example of a cartilage graft to the dorsum of the nose to correct a 'bottom heavy' nose:

a. pre-operative view
b. six months post-operatively
c. moderate tip prominence
d. six months post-operatively showing improved proportion by dorsal onlay conchal graft and slight lowering of tip.

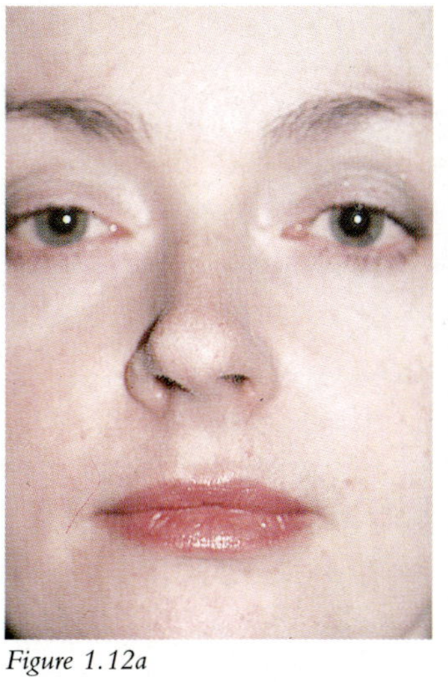

Figure 1.12a

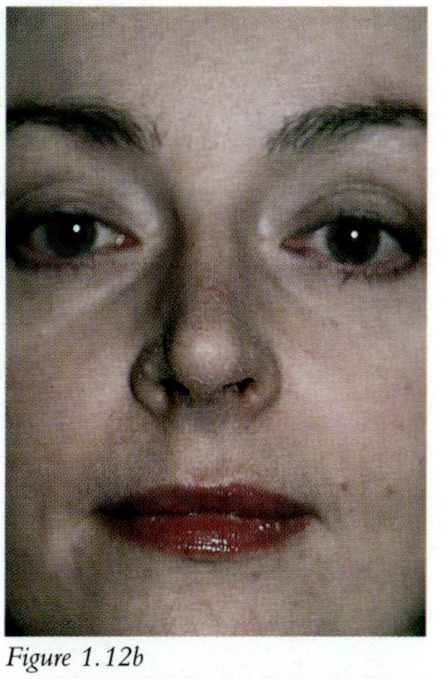

Figure 1.12b

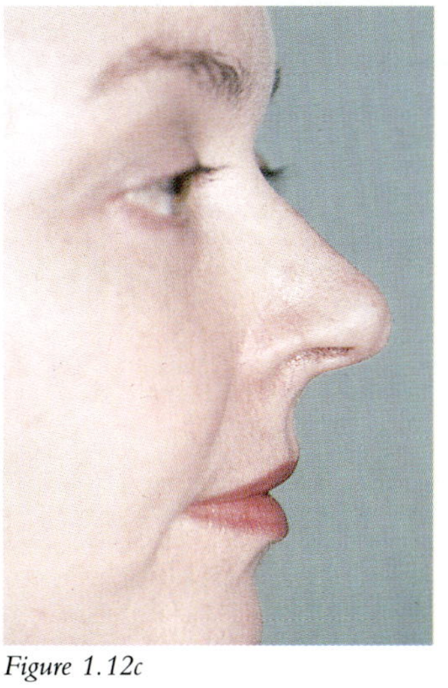

Figure 1.12c

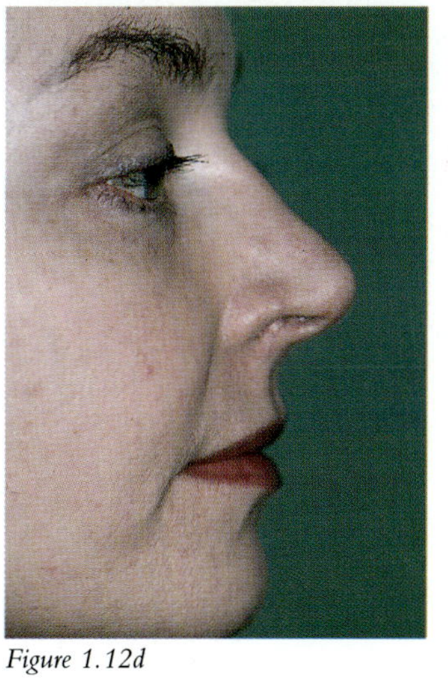

Figure 1.12d

Consultation

Selection of patients

The ability to evaluate patients undoubtedly improves through clinical experience, and for the practising plastic surgeon it is largely a matter of intuitive judgement.

This explains why some surgeons are constantly experiencing problems in their patient selection whereas others seem to have little difficulty. Today more than ever we must be on our guard against the risk of litigation; for this reason careful patient selection, good records and thoughtful patient care have become increasingly important. The less experienced surgeon is advised to read the introductory chapters to more extensive textbooks of plastic surgery where the importance of patient behaviour, psychiatric evaluation and body image are so well described.

Planning surgery

A patient's suitability for elective rhinoplasty can usually be determined at the first consultation, but detailed planning and a clear understanding of the patient make a second consultation shortly before surgery a wise routine.

A personally composed information leaflet is given to the patient at the end of the first consultation. This can then be read and familiarized before the next meeting.

I arrange for the patient to be photographed before the first consultation. These are half-plate black and white photographs, with frontal lighting and a dark background. Both lateral views, and frontal and basal views can then be examined and analysed with the patient. Tracing of one or both lateral views with suggested correction of the nasal profile is done with the patient present, as this will assist the patient's understanding and objective analysis of the problem. At this time other areas of disproportion, such as the chin,

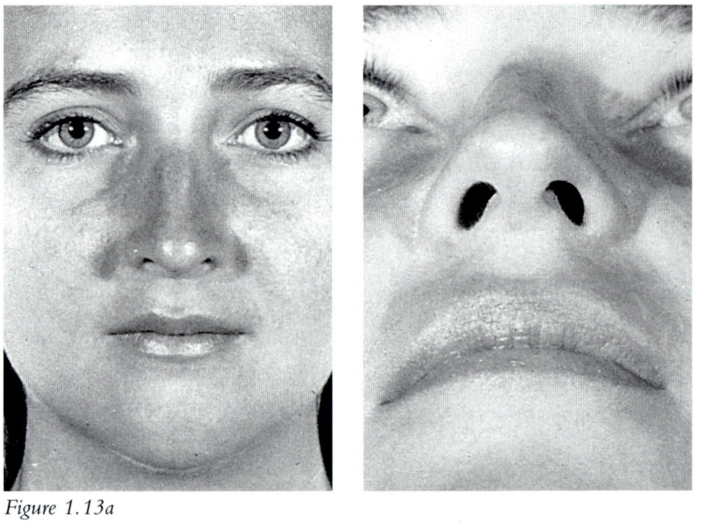

Figure 1.13a

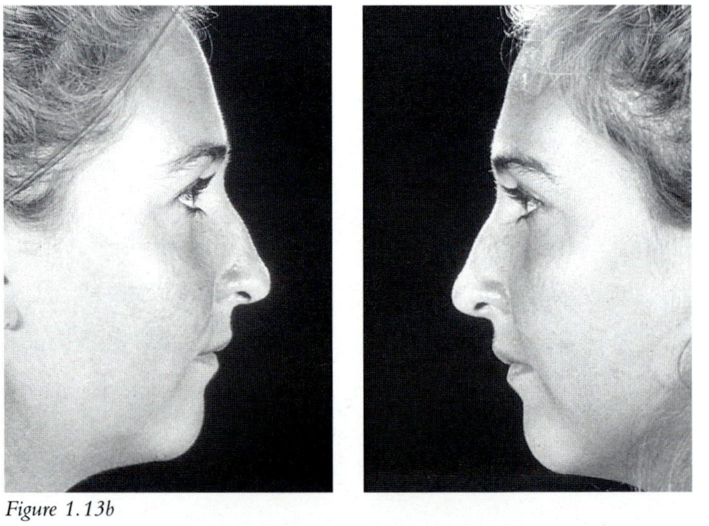

Figure 1.13b

may also be included in the discussion and drawings.

A computerized image analyser is preferred by some surgeons, but is less indicative of the surgeon's real skills; the ability to draw is a discipline that all aesthetic surgeons should learn and indeed come to enjoy. Forty years ago it was common practice to obtain a plaster mask which then allowed the surgeon to study the disproportion and correct this in three dimensions. In much the same way the image analyser allows the surgeon to measure length and angles from which to calculate the ideal proportions. Such exercises are undoubtedly beneficial to the learning curve of all practitioners and assist in the development of a higher aesthetic appreciation.

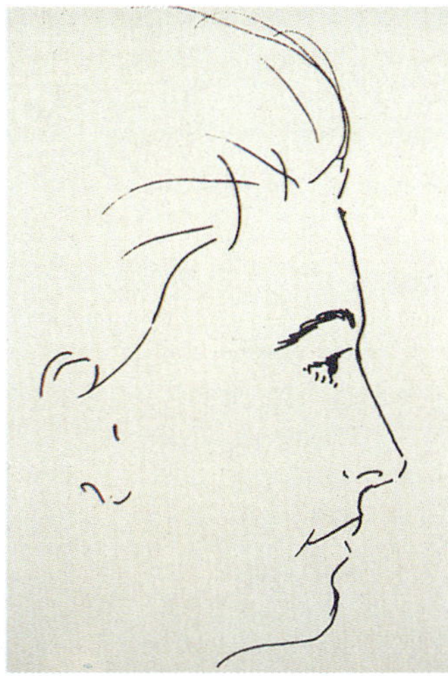

Figure 1.14

Conclusion

Rhinoplasty is an area that can be fraught with litigation; in addition, the uncertainty of the healing process means that there is a need for revisionary surgery in 7 – 10% of cases. Clear understanding and trust, developed through adequate preoperative consultations and evidence of careful documentation, will often preserve a good relationship with a disappointed patient.

It can be helpful to show and discuss these details with the patient to explain if there is any need for some secondary procedure.

If any cases reach litigation these notes will again provide weighty evidence of the careful judgement and information that the patient has received.

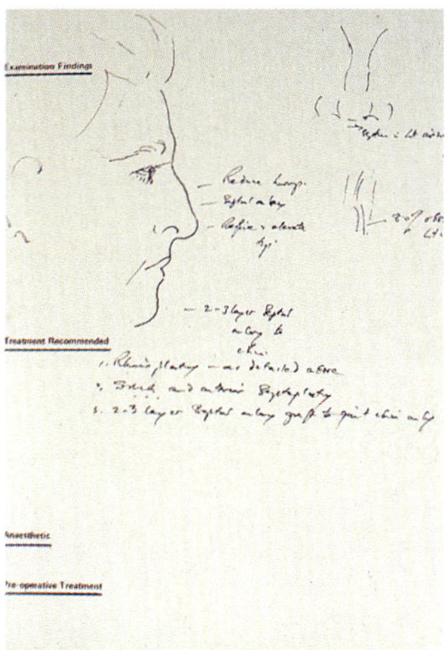

Figure 1.15

References

Edwards B. *Drawing on the Right Side of the Brain*. Los Angeles: JP Torcher Inc., 1989.

Hogarth B. *Drawing the Human Head*. New York: Watson – Guptill Publications, 1989.

Rees T. *Aesthetic Plastic Surgery*. Philadelphia: WB Saunders, 1980.

Clinics in Plastic Surgery. January 1988, **15**: 1. WB Saunders.

Clinics in Plastic Surgery. Facial Aesthetic Surgery. October 1987. **14**: 4. WB Saunders.

Part II

Basic Rhinoplasty

Mentoplasty

Basic Rhinoplasty

General anaesthesia

For most routine cases general anaesthesia is preferred with moderate hypotension combined with local infiltration of 5 – 10 ml 0.5% lignocaine : adrenaline 1 : 200 000 mixed with an equal volume and concentration of Marcaine. A nasal pack of 1 inch ribbon gauze moistened in 10% aqueous cocaine hydrochloride is inserted by the anaesthetist and removed intraoperatively before any septal surgery.

Local anaesthesia

This may be preferred when an experienced anaesthetist is not available, when performing only a partial rhinoplasty or if requested by the patient.

Preoperative sedation with promethazine hydrochloride (Phenergan) 25 mg p.o. and diazepam (Valium) 10 mg p.o. is given one hour before the operation.

In the operating room, intravenous diazepam (Diazemuls) is given in increments until speech is slurred (usually 10 – 15 mg) and then 30 – 50 mg ketamine. Blood pressure, pulse and oximeter recordings are monitored. A trance-like sedation is apparent within 1 minute which then allows time to infiltrate the nasal skin and mucosal lining with local anaesthetic.

Infiltrate the soft tissues using a 24 gauge needle, first at the nasal dome and along the dorsum, next at the nostril bases and anterior nasal spine, and then at the pyriform aperture. Advance the needle subcutaneously along the side of the dorsum up to the glabella.

Using a 30 gauge needle infiltrate a small volume subcutaneously around the region of the tip cartilages. This is an area of maximum sensibility but injection will also facilitate the submucosal dissection.

It is important to infiltrate the septal mucosa in the area of any proposed septal surgery, and also high up under the nasal bones (to obtain a dry field). Here the mucosa is thick and spongy and permits easy injection.

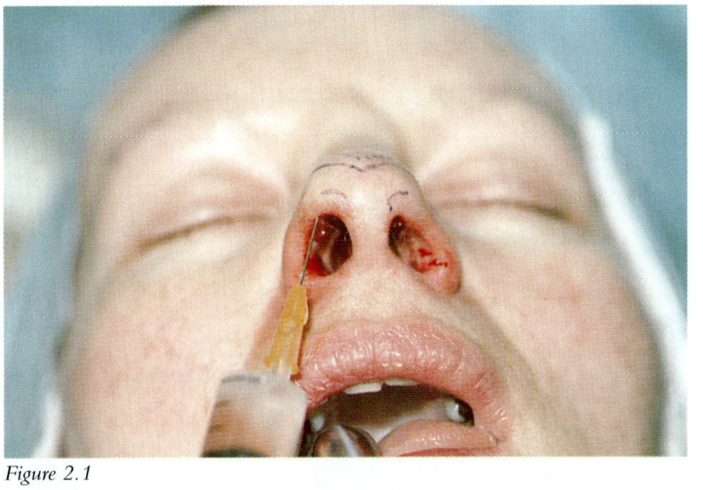

Figure 2.1

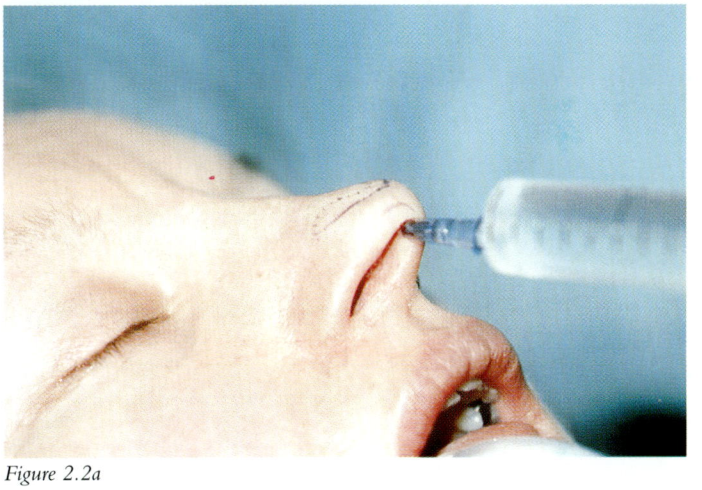

Figure 2.2a

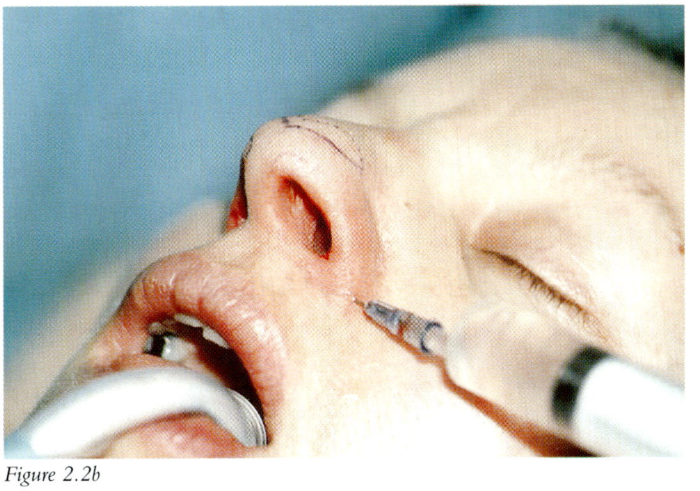

Figure 2.2b

Nasal packing with 1 inch ribbon gauze moistened in a 10% aqueous solution of cocaine hydrochloride gives further anaesthesia, particularly in the posterior nasal structures and turbinates; it is also of value if using local anaesthesia, because it checks any bleeding that would otherwise run posteriorly and induce coughing.

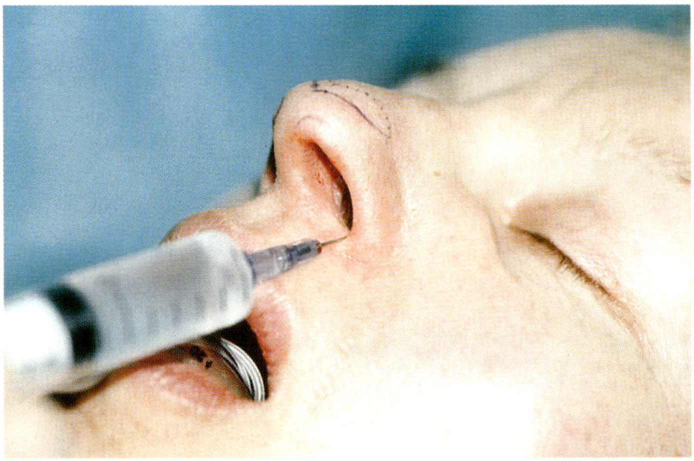

Figure 2.2c

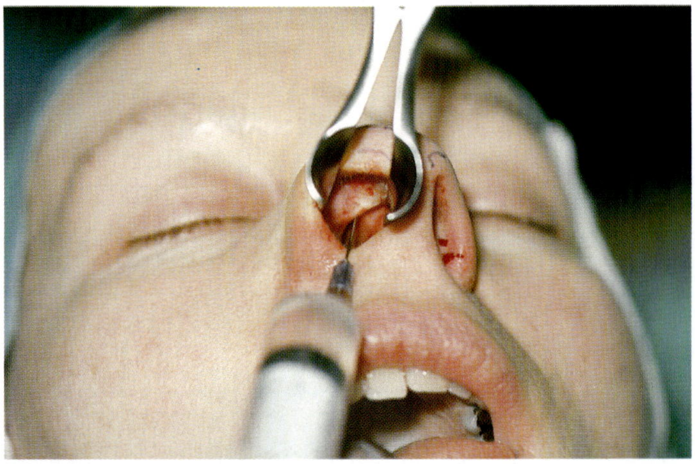

Figure 2.3

Incisions

Clean the vestibules of any crusts and shave the vibrissi with a no. 15 scalpel. This is simpler and more efficient than scissors. However, when secondary deformity or scar contractures cause irregularity a more painstaking trimming with scissors may be unavoidable.

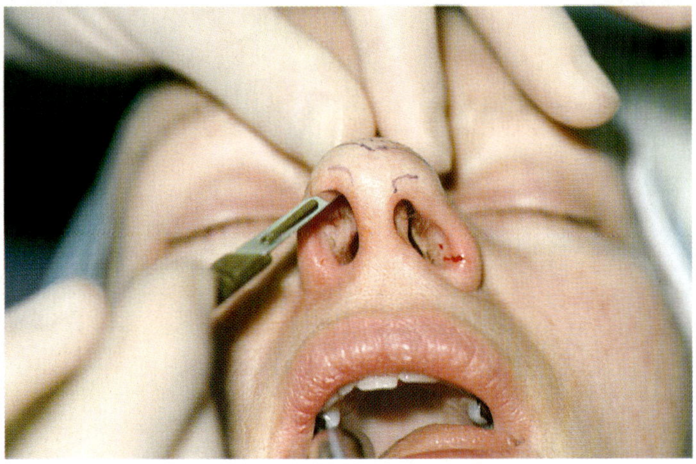

Figure 2.4

Skin markings

These are both an important guide and a preliminary step in planning surgery.

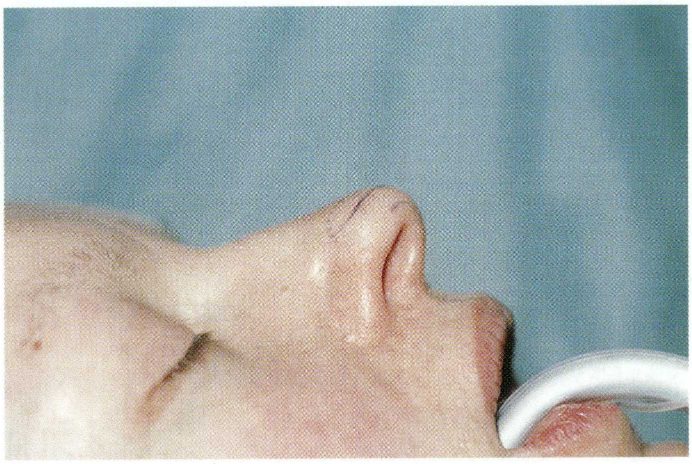

Figure 2.5

The size and firmness (thickness) of the tip cartilages will influence the amount removed.

Fig 2.6a Excess alar base excision will result from this incision.

Fig 2.6b Excess tip excision will result from this incision.

Fig 2.6c Preservation of correct amount of al;ar cartilage in tip and full length of lateral crus.

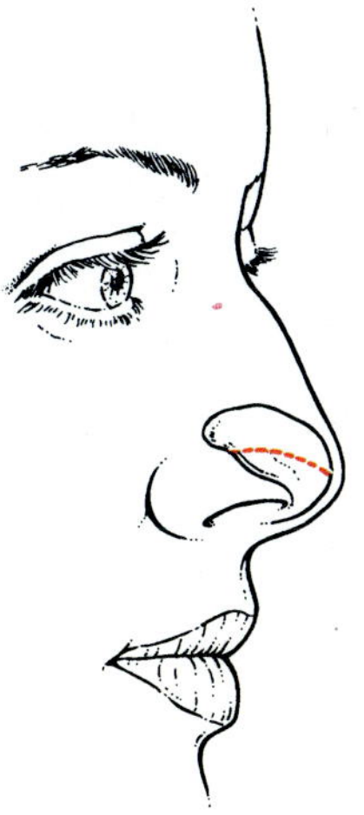

Figure 2.6a

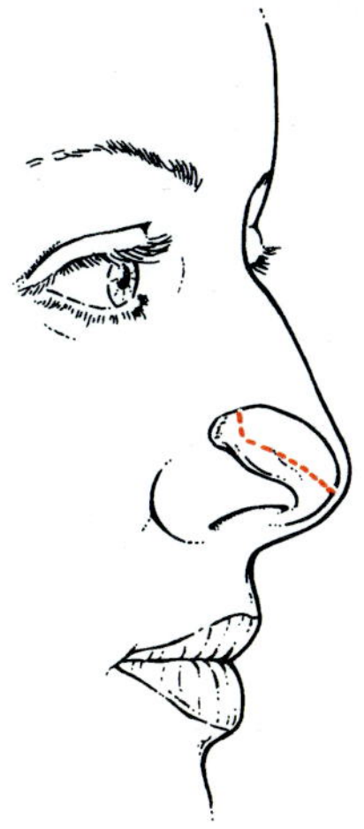

Figure 2.6b

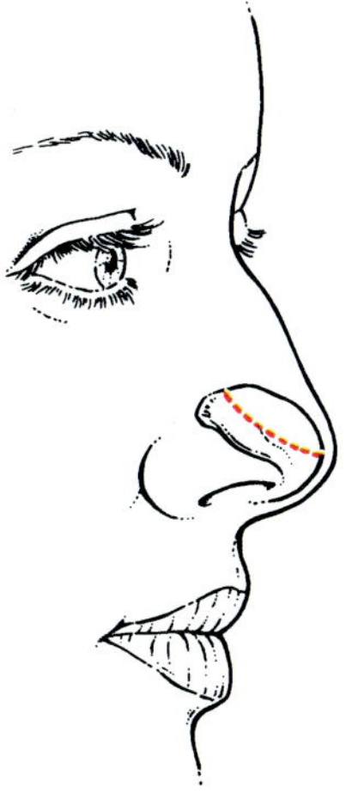

Figure 2.6c

When the cartilage is thin and pliable, remove much less of the lateral crus, otherwise too much tip projection will be lost or a pinched tip with excessive alar grooves may develop postoperatively.

Transcartilaginous incision

Eversion of the nostril rim with a thimble retractor causes the skin to blanche along the caudal border, enabling the surgeon to make an incision parallel to this and usually at a distance of 4 – 5 mm. Counterpressure from the finger tip overlying the skin marking is a further guide to the exact level of this incision. The incision is now made through the nasal skin and underlying lateral crus of the vestibule, curving this in a cephalic direction, so that the full width of the lateral crus is preserved towards its outer third.

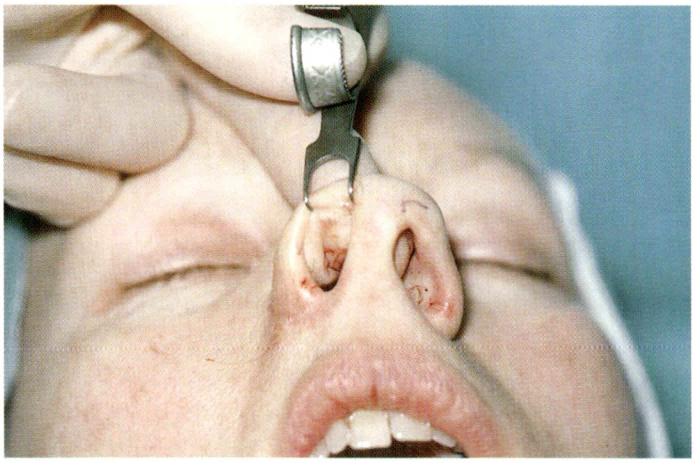

Figure 2.7

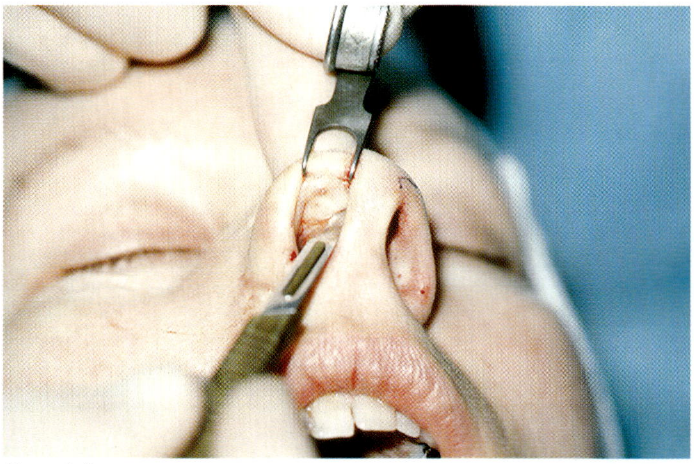

Figure 2.8

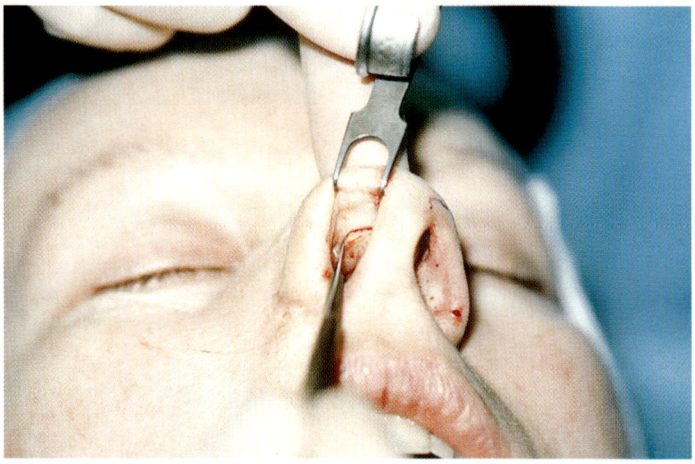

Figure 2.9

Repeat this on the opposite side and then join the two by a transfixation incision through the membranous portion of the septum.

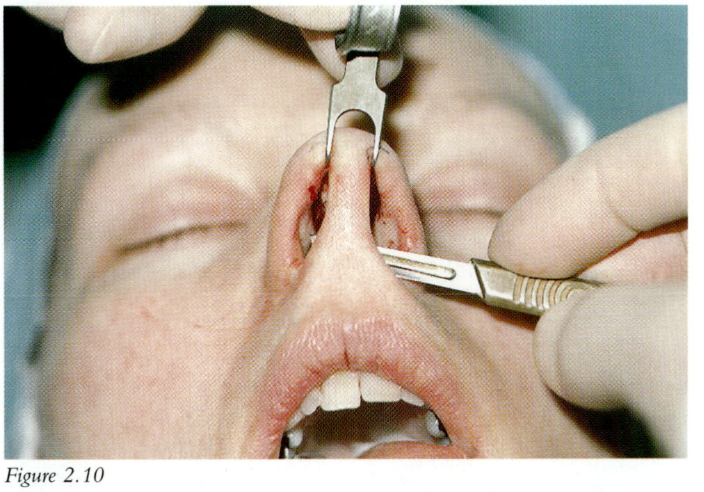

Figure 2.10

Remember that additional lateral crus can always be trimmed through the same incision, so when in doubt be conservative. Minimal cartilage removal is often sufficient and will give a pleasing refinement to the tip.

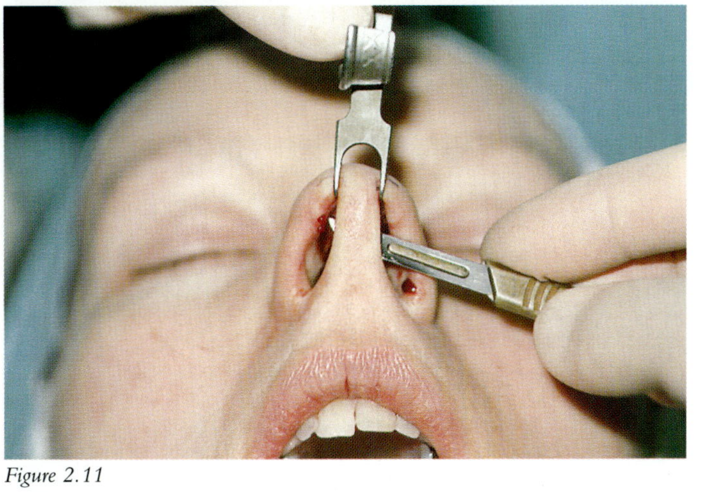

Figure 2.11

Removal of excess lateral crus

This is conveniently done now while the same exposure is maintained with the finger tip (left hand) and thimble retractor.

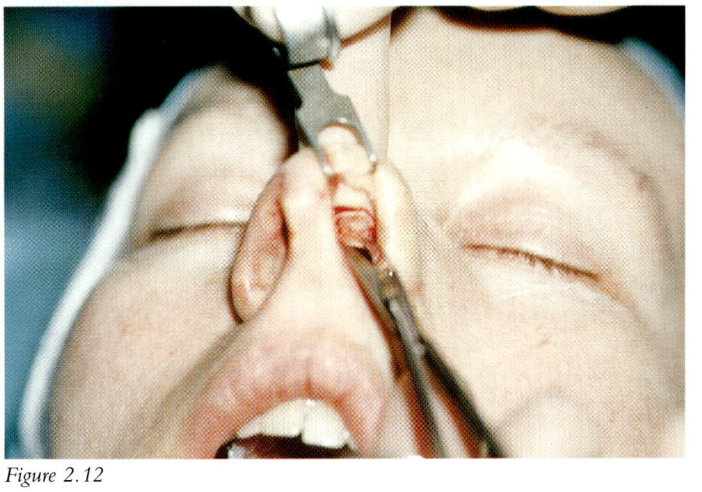

Figure 2.12

Gently insert the tip of the curved iris scissors between the nasal mucosa and cartilage and then spread the blades apart. The cartilage is fragile and care must be taken as the mucosa is adherent to it.
Separation of the outer surface is easy in contrast, because attachment to the fibrofatty areola tissues is loose.
The assistant now takes the thimble retractor and the surgeon can complete division and removal of the dissected portion of the lateral crus, still attached laterally and medially.

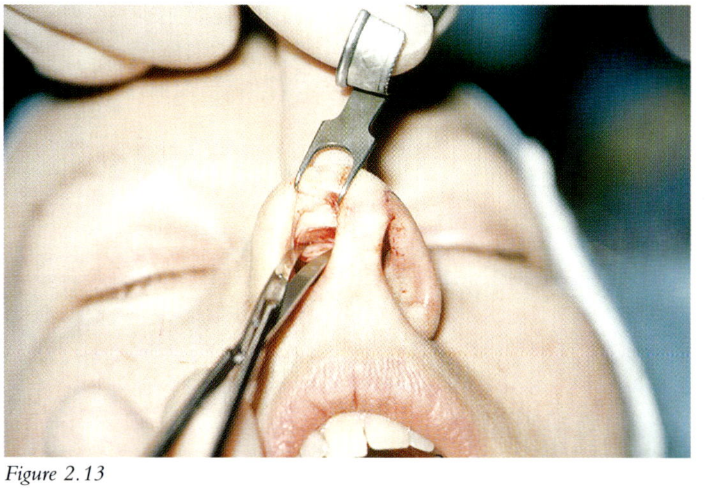
Figure 2.13

Grasp the mid-portion of the cartilage with tooth forceps and complete separation with the same scissors.
This preliminary tip cartilage dissection gives access to the nasal dorsum and is therefore a logical first step. I now prefer to complete the dorsal surgery and then return to the tip surgery as a final stage when delicate adjustment to the height and width of the tip and to the columella give the ultimate effect.

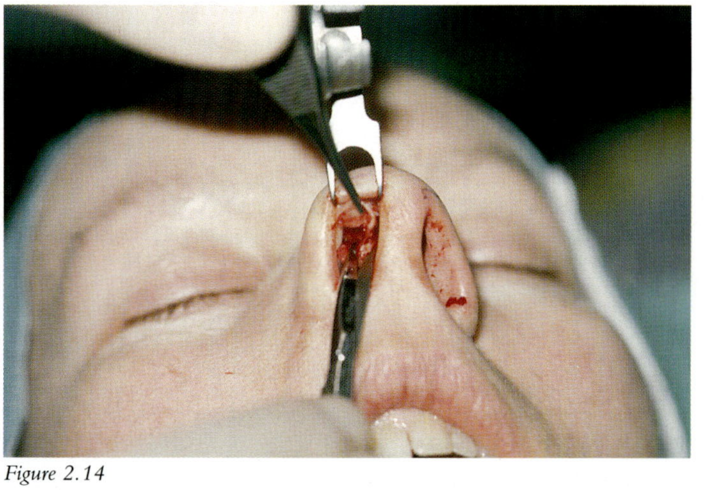
Figure 2.14

Dorsum of the nose
Undermining of the dorsum is carried out subperiosteally because this preserves the soft tissues and avoids, in particular, any scarring in the subcutaneous adipose layer.

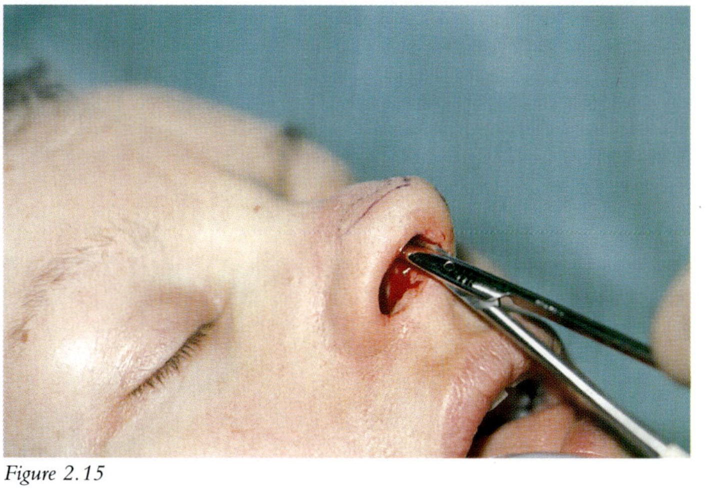
Figure 2.15

Extend the dissection with scissors to the pyriform margins; then insert a Joseph periosteal elevator along the outer margin of the proposed area of undermining.

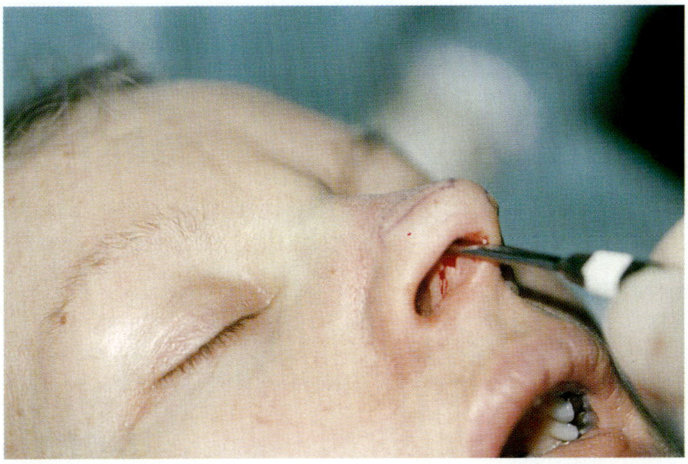

Figure 2.16

With sideways movements strip the periosteum up to the mid-line, after which do the same on the opposite side; then join across the mid-line.

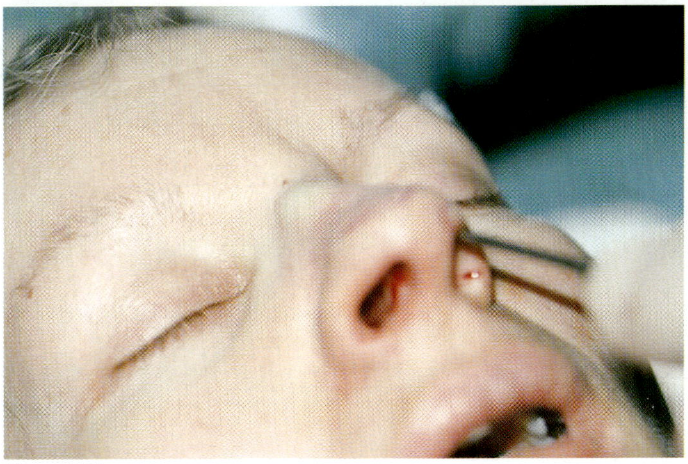

Figure 2.17

It is not necessary to undermine widely, the aim being to allow sufficient space for the skin to adapt smoothly following hump removal.

The smaller the hump, the less skin undermining is required.

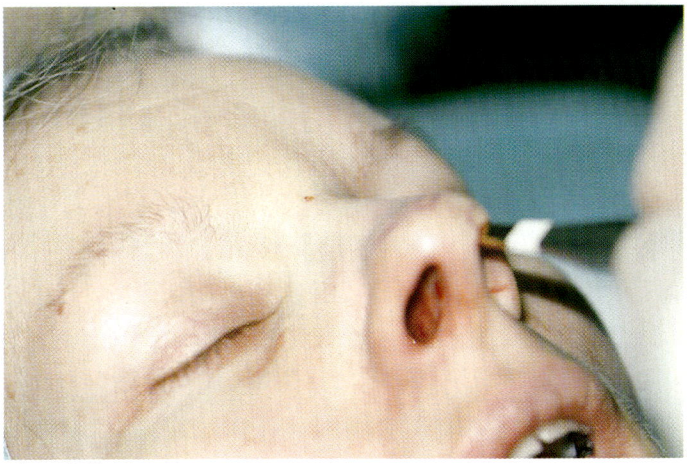

Figure 2.18

Removal of the dorsal bony hump

For the inexperienced surgeon the saw or osteotome can lead to inaccurate and excessive removal, and undoubtedly modern rhinoplasty rasps, for example, as made by Snowden Penser, are the safest technique for the beginner.

With experience, the saw offers a more sophisticated method for cleanly incising the bone, with less risk of damage to the upper lateral cartilages and preservation of the hump for possible use as a graft. The newer saws are finer and sharper, such as those made by Stortz and Snowden Penser, which are my personal preference.

Make the saw cut initially on the side opposite to the surgeon, with the left index finger providing stability and guidance. The cut extends only through the bone to the midline (and not the upper lateral cartilages). Now complete the cut from the right side.

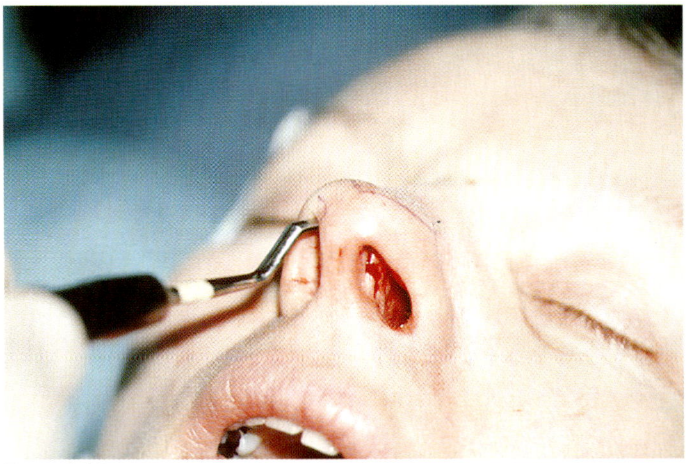

Figure 2.19

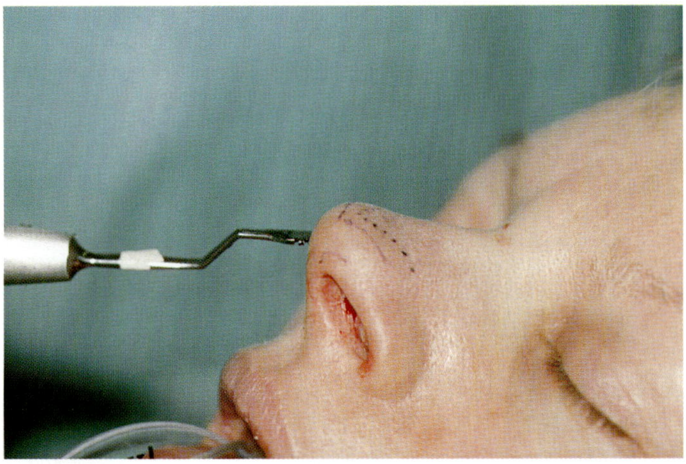

Figure 2.20

For minimal bony hump removal I generally use the saw, using it as a lateral cutting rasp because this leaves clean-cut edges to the bony dorsum.
The saw is therefore a convenient instrument for removal of even the smallest hump.

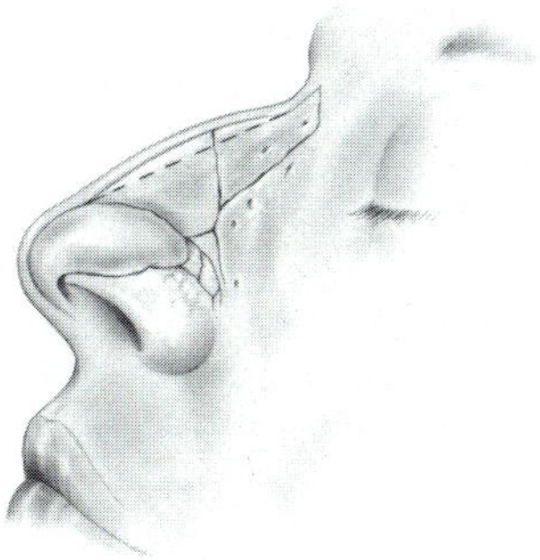

Figure 2.21

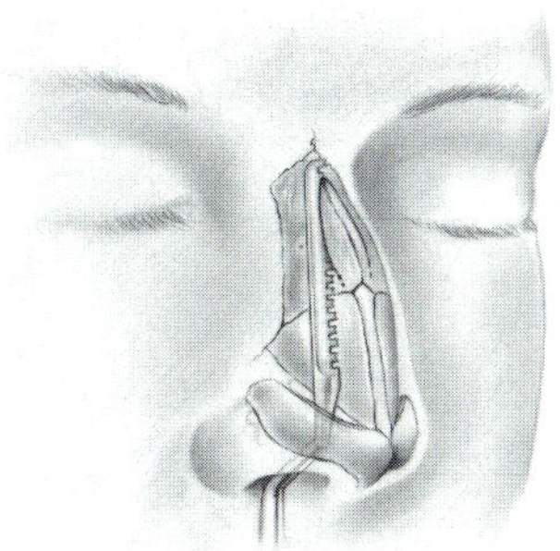

Figure 2.22

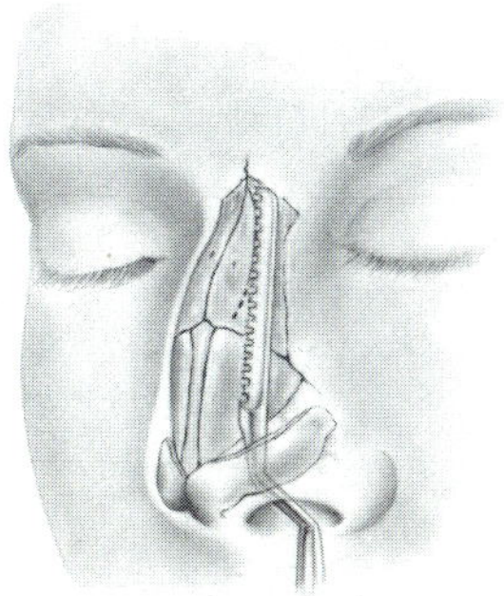

Figure 2.23

Removal of the cartilaginous hump
This is done using a no. 11 scalpel blade with the sharp point first broken off.

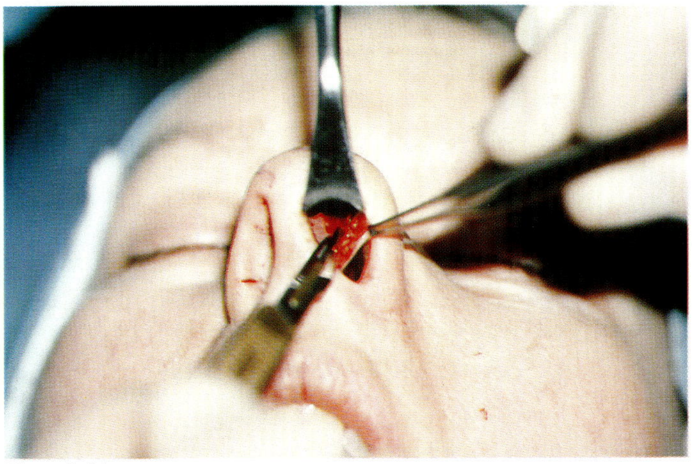

Figure 2.24

Extramucosal incision is desirable. Apply gentle traction with forceps to the caudal border of the septal mucosa, at the same time dissecting the mucosa off the undersurface of the cartilaginous vault with the no. 11 scalpel.

The amount of stripping will be dependent on the size of the hump to be removed, but 0.5 cm is sufficient for minor and moderate hump excisions. The mucosa is now preserved intact in the region of the internal valve.

Introduce the no. 11 scalpel into the saw cut and, with the nostril rim safely retracted (using an Aufricht retractor), shave down the septum and upper lateral cartilages by the appropriate amount. Be conservative because further reduction can easily be done with a further cut if necessary.

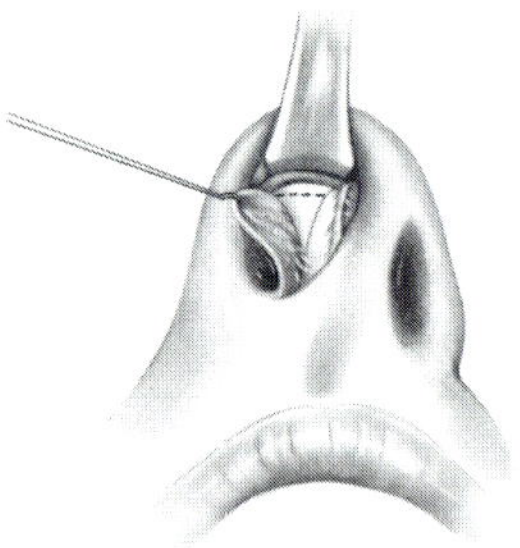

Figure 2.25

Further refinements

Bony dorsum Using a nasal rasp chamfer the sharp bony cut surface into a smooth curve, and at the same time smooth off the anterior angle of the nasal bones. The two manoeuvres are especially important when the nasal bones are thick, because in this way a smooth gradation from bony to cartilaginous dorsum is produced.

Cartilaginous dorsum Make the initial cut cautiously because secondary lesser trimming of a millimetre or more may be required, especially at the anterior angle. Final adjustment is also made near completion of the rhinoplasty when all other components have been adjusted.

Lateral osteotomy Incise the mucosa at the pyriform aperture with a no. 15 blade. Raise a subperiosteal tunnel with a Joseph elevator along the base of the frontal process of the maxilla. Use a guarded 4 mm osteotome for the osteotomy. Make sure the cut is started at the base of the pyriform aperture so that there is no palpable step following infracture. The right hand holds the chisel firmly, the

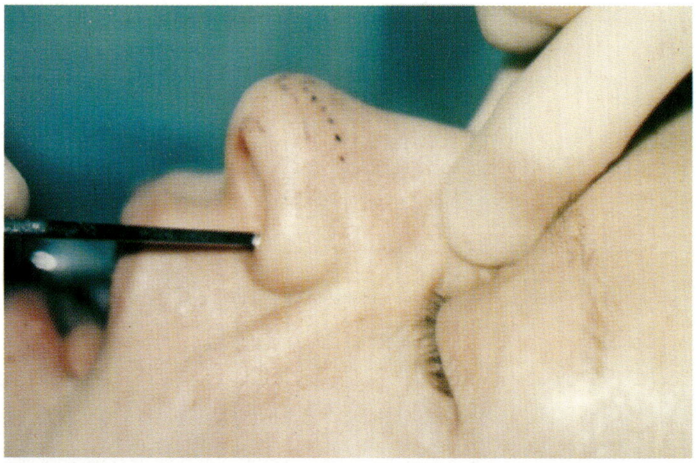

Figure 2.26

left index finger palpates the leading edge of the osteotome as it advances, and the assistant operates the hammer.

The osteotomy follows the angle between the cheek and bony dorsum, curving medially over the cephalic portion until resistance is reached and a duller percussion sound heard. A gentle upward (anterior) elevation of the handle of the osteotome by a few degrees, or medial rotation of the osteotome, completes the osteotomy especially in the younger or female patient in whom the bones are either more flexible or thinner. In cases of removal of a very small hump the bony dorsum will remain intact over the nasion, and must be separated before attempting infracture.

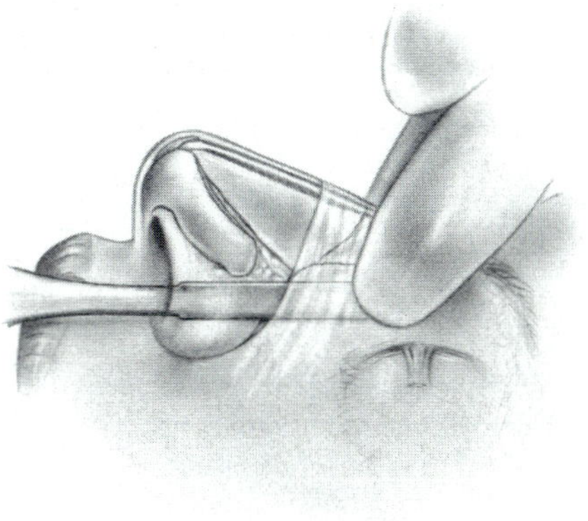

Figure 2.27

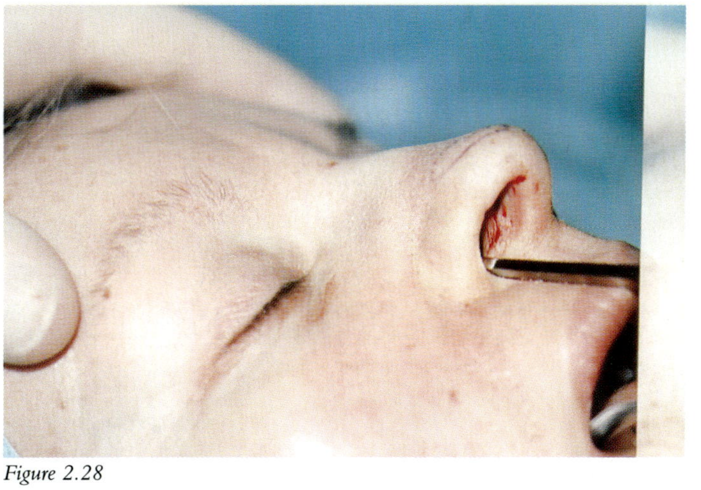

Figure 2.28

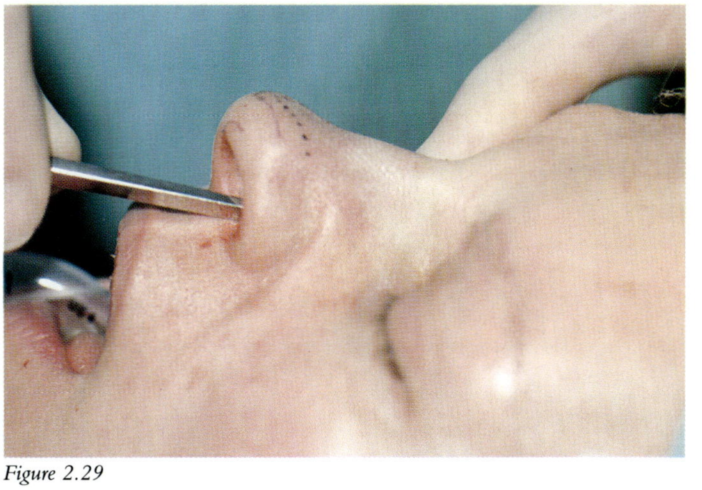

Figure 2.29

To complete the osteotomy introduce the curved osteotome along the saw cut, angling it downwards (posteriorly) 20° and slightly laterally.

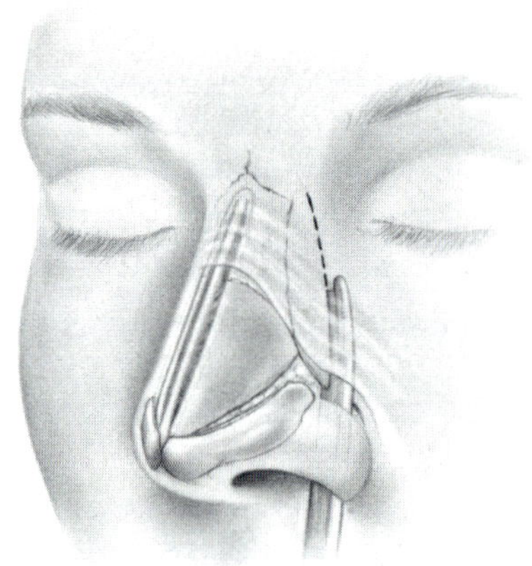

Figure 2.30

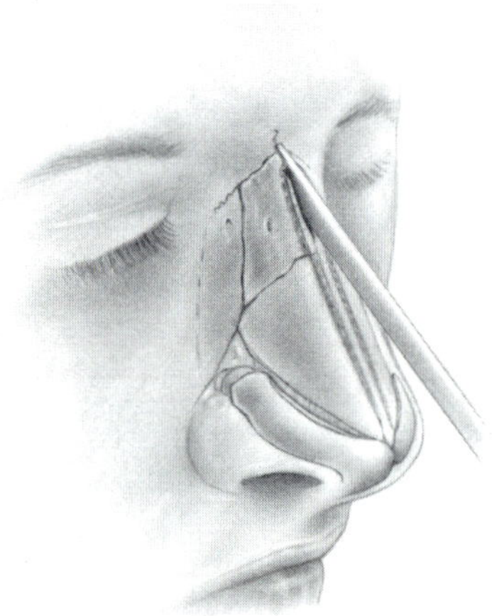

Figure 2.31

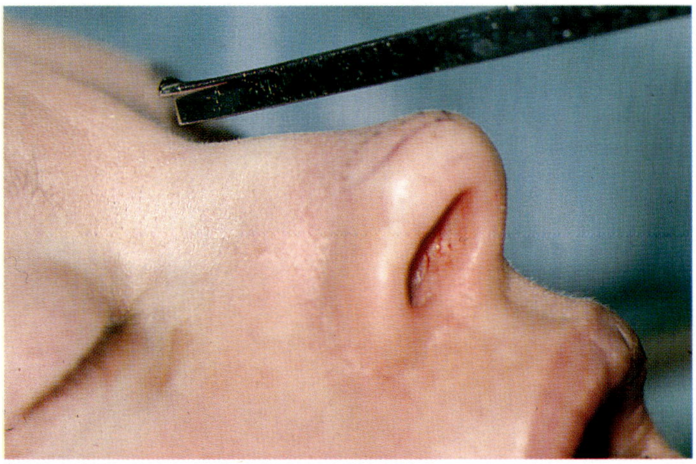

Figure 2.32

A gentle tap with the hammer will complete the bony separation. This is then repeated on the opposite side.

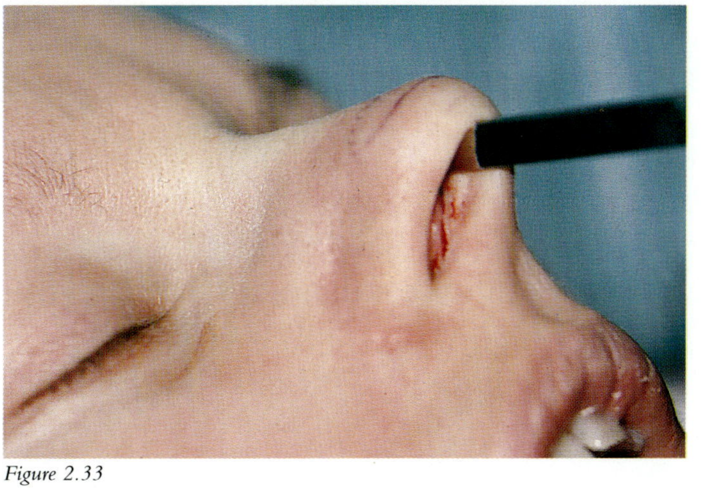

Figure 2.33

Additional procedures

1. *In older patients* with hard brittle bones, and especially in those with thick nasal bones, there is a risk of fracturing the nasal bones at too caudal a level. In these cases it is safer to perform a preliminary partial osteotomy with nasal saw, and then complete it in the usual manner with the curved osteotome.

2. *A wide bony dorsum*, thick nasal bones, or those with more pronounced divergence of the nasal bones, have a web of bone at the cephalic end of the hump removal.

This can either cause the nasal bones to fracture at the wrong level or can block approximation of the bones after osteotomy. It is important to remove this bony web following hump removal and before infracture, and this is most easily done by gentle vertical saw cuts with the nasal saws.

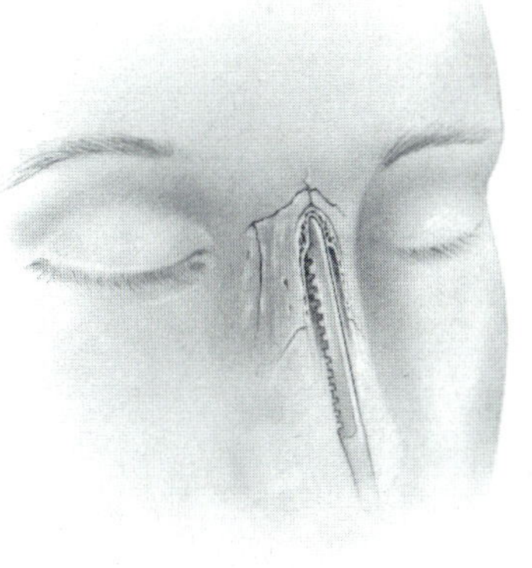

Figure 2.34

Minimal resistance is first encountered; continue sawing until resistance is felt against the thick glabellar bone. It is at this level that completion of the osteotomy with an osteotome may become necessary as already described.

Osteotomy at a more cephalic level is undesirable and can lead to 'see-sawing' of the nasal bones, with unwanted prominence of the glabellar bone when the mid-third of the dorsum is narrowed.

Supra tip

In the region from which tip cartilage was removed, there is usually an excess of underlying fibrofatty tissue, which is now removed, otherwise this tissue will contribute postoperatively to an undesirable supratip hump or soft tissue excess.

Insert the tip scissors through the transcartilaginous incision with the scissor tip towards the tip of the nose and the jaws open.

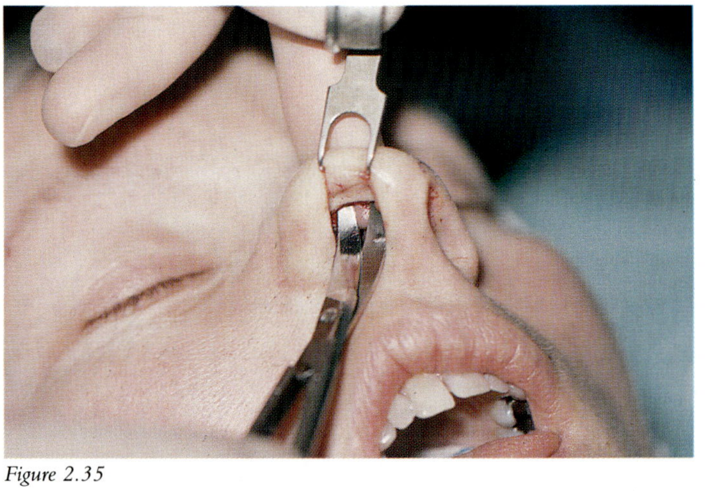

Figure 2.35

Light counterpressure with the finger tip of the opposite hand will then push the excess fat into the opened scissors, and facilitate excision.

In this way the fibrofatty tissue is usually removed in three to four small pieces.

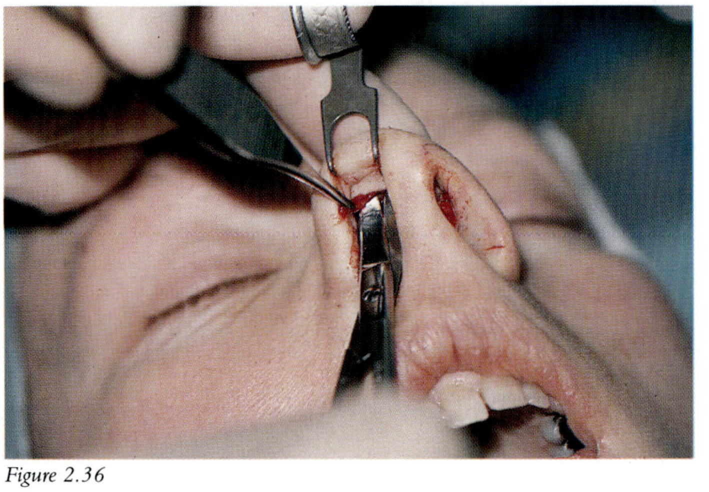

Figure 2.36

Nasal tip

The remaining portion of the lateral crura and the dome are tightly adherent to overlying skin, and are now partly undermined with the tip scissors.

This should be done just enough to allow the overlying skin to accommodate more easily. For simple rhinoplasty no further tip work is needed. For high or wide tips additional manoeuvres are used, and are described on pages 59–68.

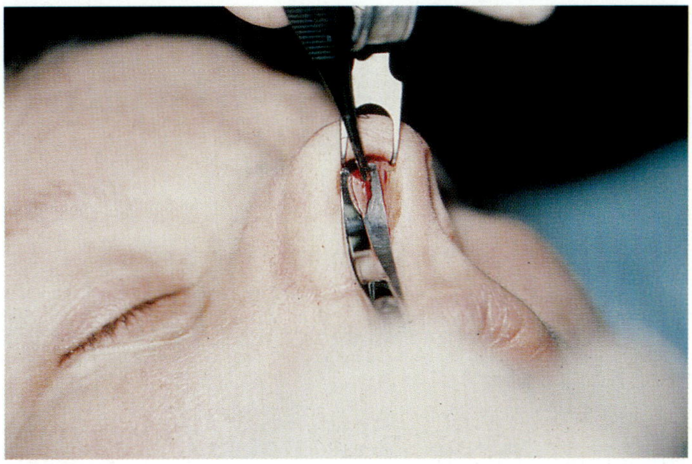

Figure 2.37

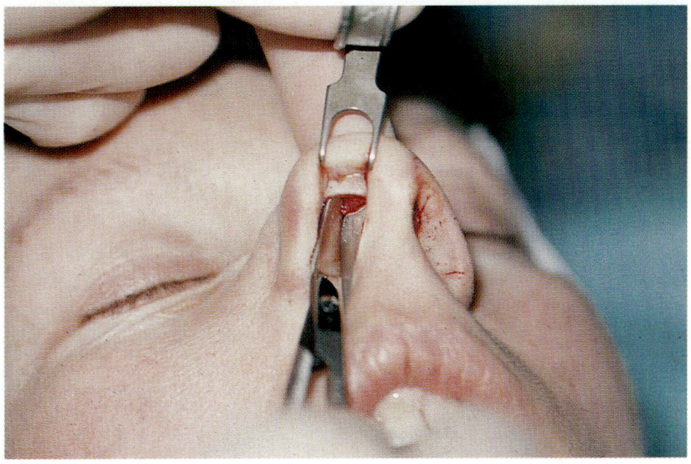

Figure 2.38

Shortening the septum and adjusting the columella

Any reduction in the nasal skeleton will produce some relaxation in the overlying soft tissue cover.

A slight compensatory shortening of the septum may be carried out by trimming of the cut surface of the membranous septum. For greater effect the cartilage is trimmed a few millimetres. The anterior one-third of the septum is bevelled to accommodate the lobular portion of the tip. More radical shortening is not usually indicated and will result in an unnaturally 'snubby nose' and longer upper lip.

With conservative tip reduction the columella will frequently accommodate without need for any adjustment.

If the tip of the nose appears too prominent as a result of too much columellar support, make a slight accommodation by releasing the soft tissues and depressor muscle attached to the anterior nasal spine.

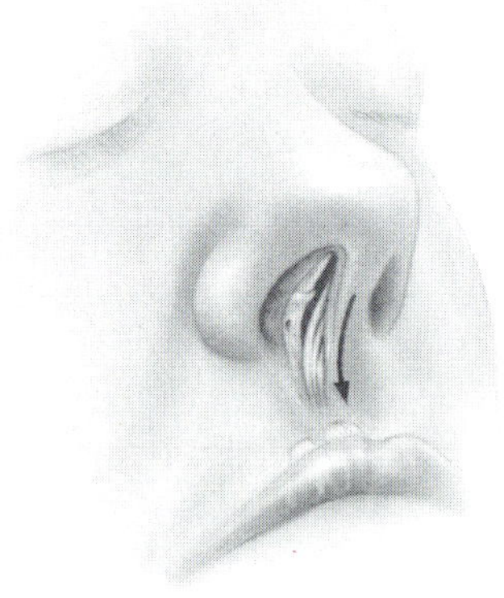

Figure 2.39

Use mainly blunt dissection with the tip scissors.

For correction of an overly long columella, see page 79.

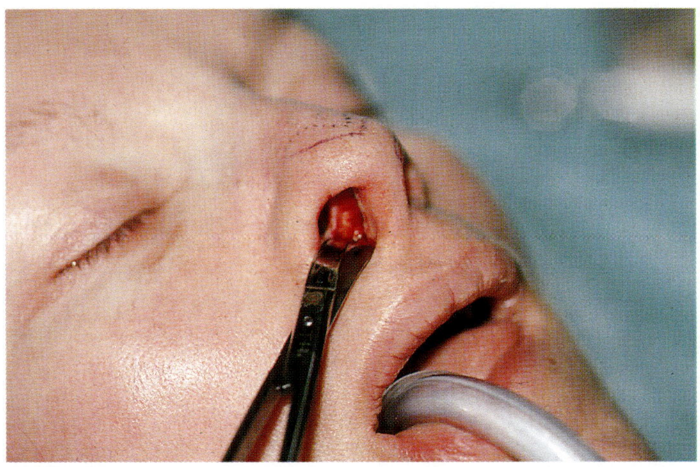

Figure 2.40

Cartilage grafts to tip and columella

Refinement of the nasal tip in primary rhinoplasty may require a small sculpted onlay tip graft inserted through a 6 – 7 mm rim incision. This will also be indicated for correction of a depressed tip.

Mark the skin of the tip to plan and define the exact location for the graft and its size.

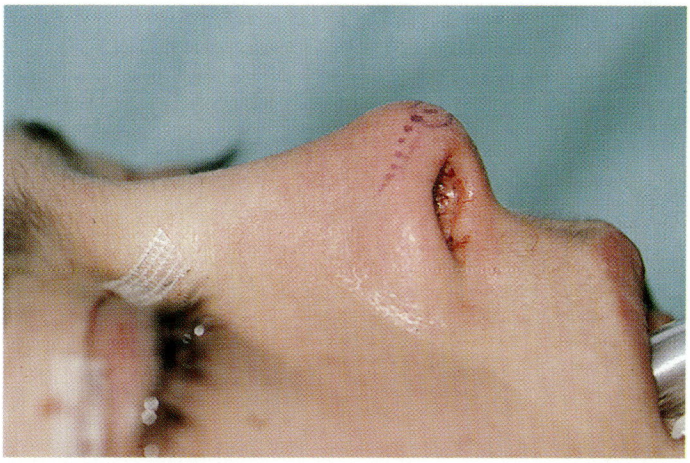

Figure 2.41

Septal cartilage is the preferred material. This is the most readily available (unless you can make use of the tip cartilage already removed).

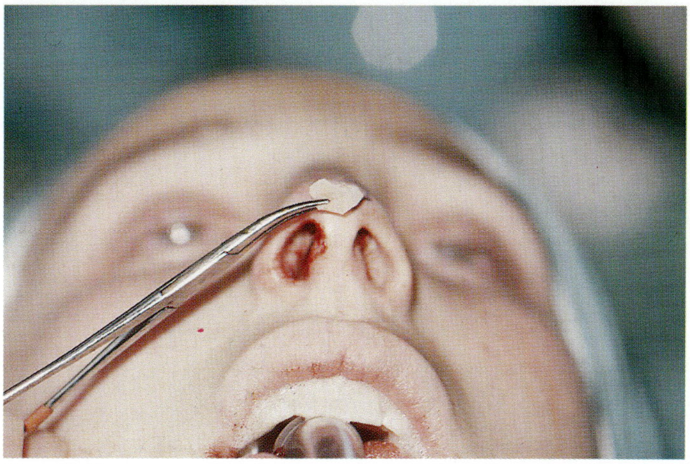

Figure 2.42

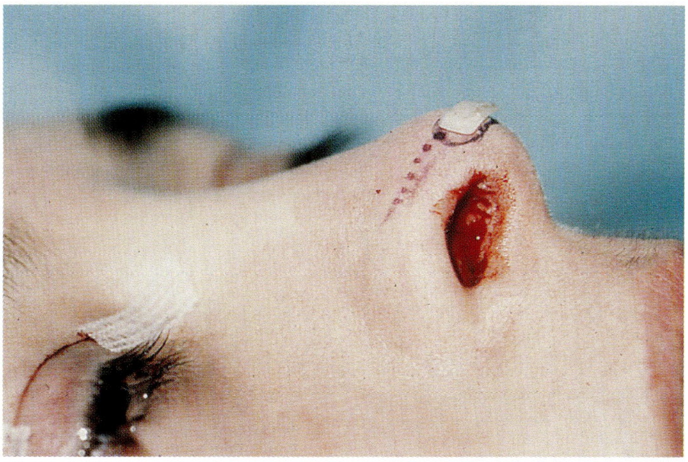

Figure 2.43

The more superficial layer (outer) graft must be finely tapered and very precisely carved to blend smoothly on to the underlying tip cartilages.

Septal cartilage is always the preferred material because it can be sculpted more precisely. Badly prepared grafts or thick conchal grafts will tend to become visible, especially when the skin of the nasal tip is thin.

Design the shape of the graft to reproduce the bifid shape of the underlying median crura and domes. A simple oval or rectangular-shaped graft does not reproduce the subtle anatomy of an attractive nasal tip and will give a less pleasing result.

Do not attempt to use a cartilage crusher to flatten septal cartilage; it will shatter into fragments. The secret of success is to take extreme care to bevel the edges finely, so that they are soft and pliable and blend naturally against the underlying tip cartilage.

In contrast conchal cartilage which is softer and less compact may be rendered flatter and limper by crushing; it cannot, however, be carved so finely. It is better suited for dorsal onlay grafts than tip grafts.

Technique

Incise just inside the nostril rim for approximately 6 – 7 mm.

Undermine the tip skin with fine dissecting scissors, making a space very slightly larger than the skin marking.

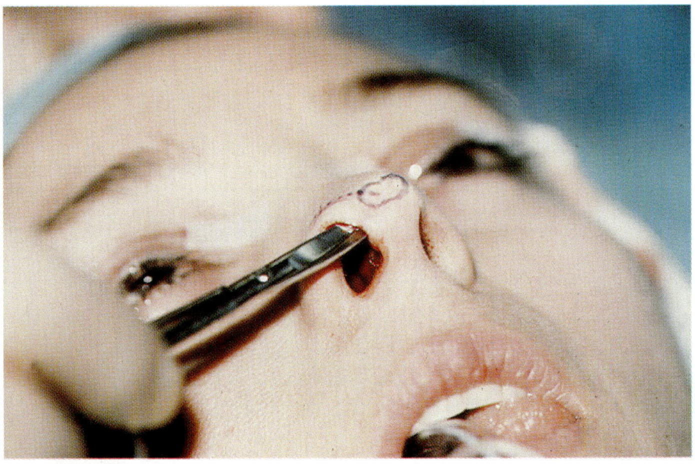

Figure 2.44

Sculpt the graft with a no. 15 scalpel taking care to bevel the edges on the outer side, so that they blend smoothly with the underlying tip cartilage.

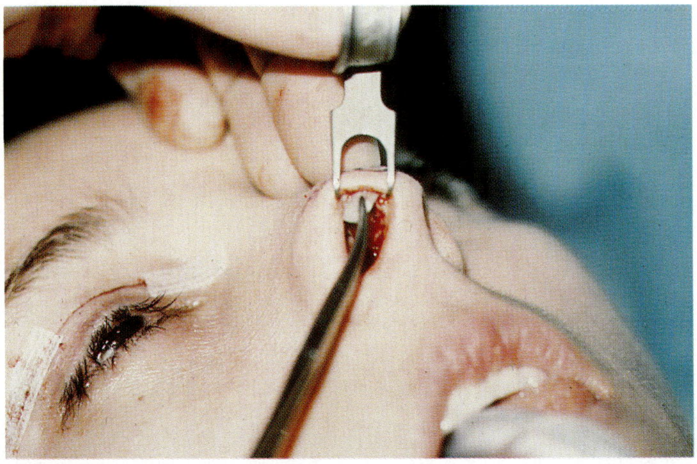

Figure 2.45

The size and shape will vary but should not exceed 8 mm in length.

A bilobular graft will give the best tip definition. Elevation of the tip may require a second layer of cartilage, but more will exaggerate the length of the lobular portion of the tip and create disproportion in relation to columellar length. A tip that is flat in profile may require the creation of a columellar-lobular angle and the Sheen type of tip graft is indicated. It is advisable to keep the vertical height of this graft slightly shorter, because any over-stretching of the lobular portion of the tip has an unnatural and unflattering appearance.

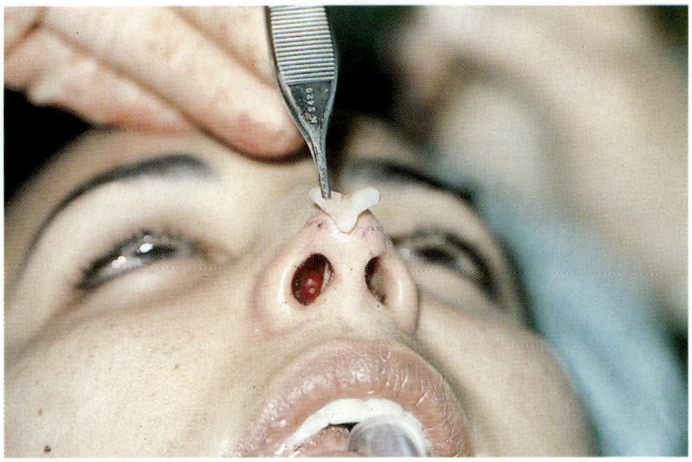

Figure 2.46

Figure 2.47 demonstrates correct level for tip graft.

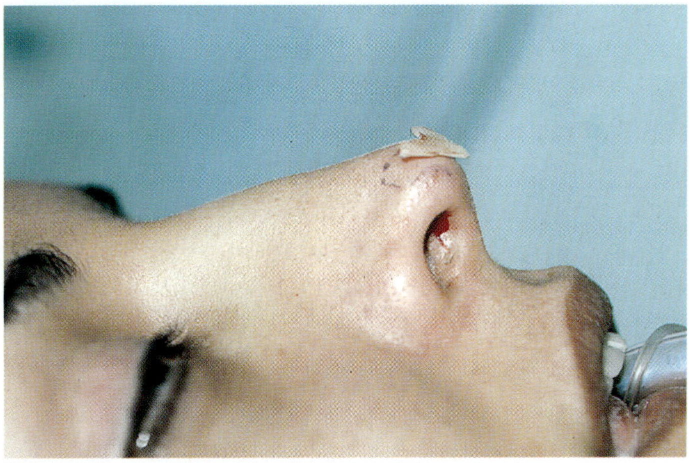

Figure 2.47

Figure 2.48 shows improved tip definition and projection after tip graft inserted.

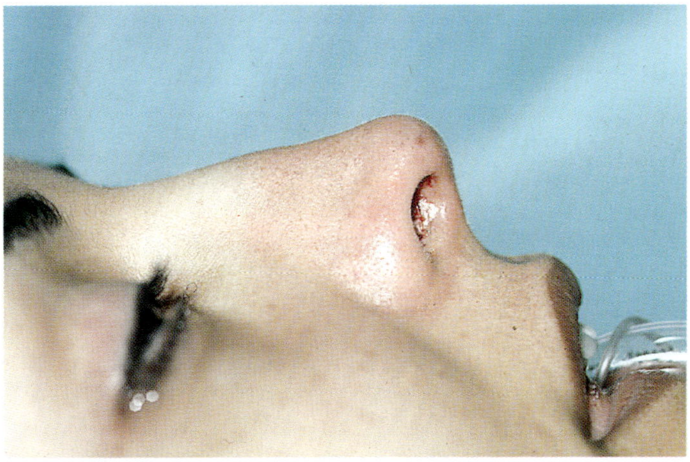

Figure 2.48

Elevation of the tip alone by onlay grafts will not produce full correction of the underlying defect. Instead a columellar strut or onlay graft to the base is required.

I prefer to insert an inverted T-shaped graft which remains stable in the mid-line and does not slip down into the lip.

Using tip scissors dissect a small space down on to the maxilla immediately anterior to the nasal spine.

Separate the medial crura within the columella using scissors but towards the tip make a tunnel instead to secure the anterior end of the graft.

The graft is cut from septal cartilage which is stiffer than conchal cartilage and less bulky, so that it does not cause undesirable fullness to the columella.

Spread the soft tissues overlying the region of the anterior nasal spine with the tip scissors. Through this slit-like opening the base of the columellar graft is inserted down on to the bone.

With the thimble retractor apply gentle traction to the nasal tip, which allows the columellar graft to slip into the tunnel in the lobular portion of the tip.

Close the skin incision in the membranous portion of the septum with a few sutures of 4.0 catgut.

A columellar strut extending into the tip should be combined with a tip graft — a Peck 'umbrella graft', because this will otherwise form an undesirable pressure point in the skin overlying the tip.

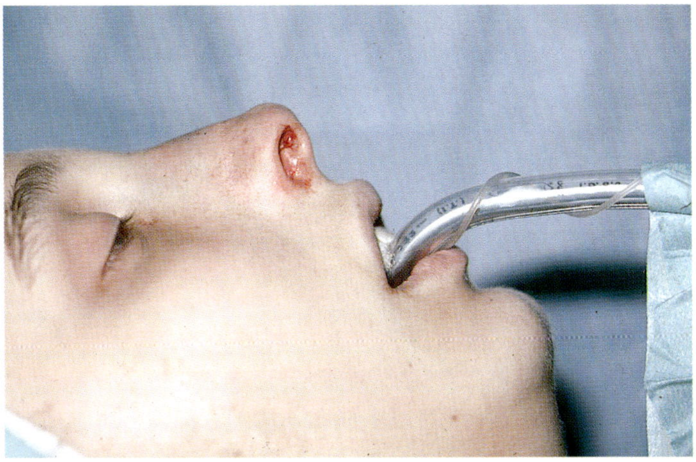

Figure 2.49

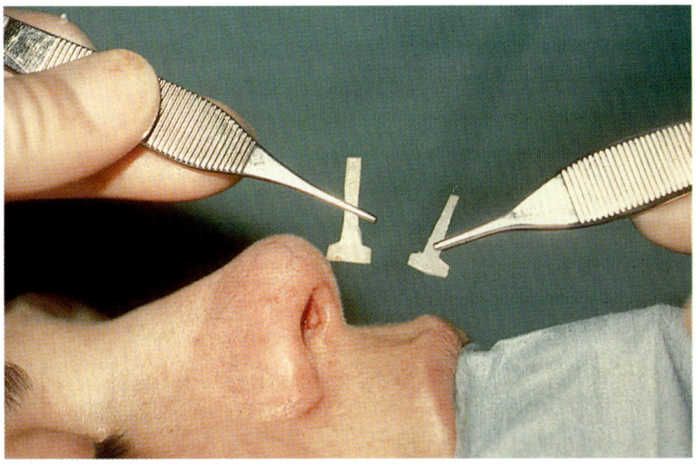

Figure 2.50

When the soft tissues are inelastic, scarred and contracted, gentle stretching will produce correction after which the graft is inserted more easily. Use the side and tip of the tip scissors to lift and stretch the soft tissues gently. Be patient and never exert more than gentle pressure.

Insert the graft into the subcutaneous pocket where it remains stable, and close the skin with two or three 6.0 plain catgut sutures.

Inadequate projection of the nasal tip may be caused by a short or unsupported columella which becomes more obvious when smiling.

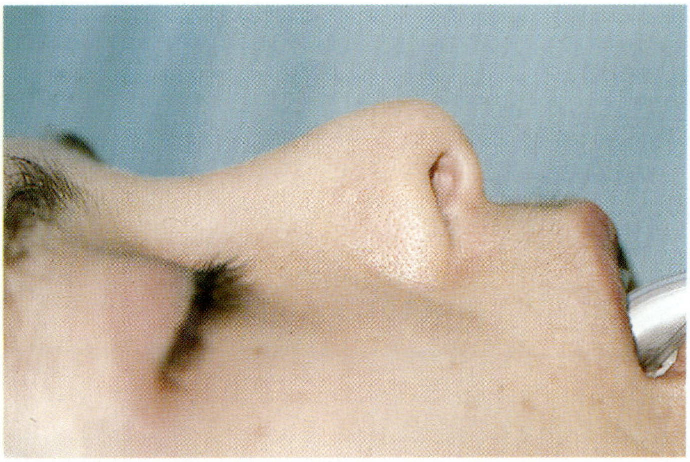

Figure 2.51

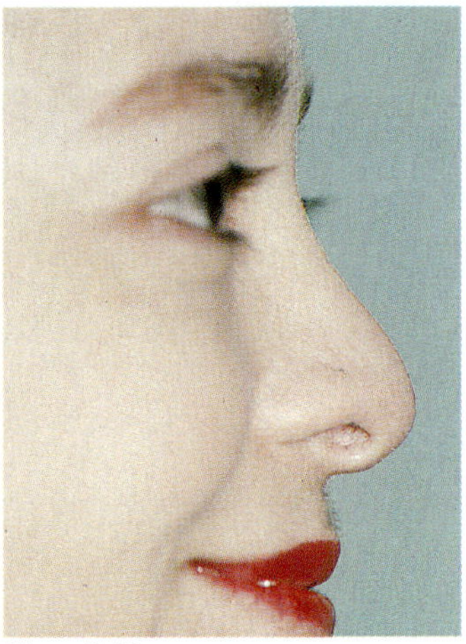

Figure 2.52

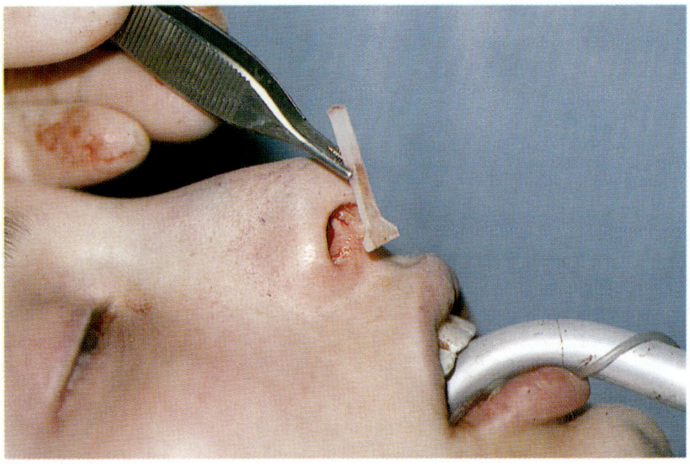

Figure 2.53

Figures 2.53 and 2.54 show improved tip projection in which columellar strut as well as tip graft are necessary.

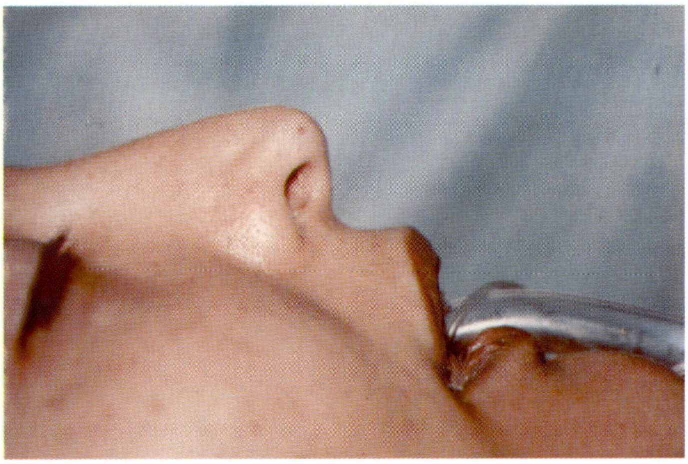

Figure 2.54

A T-shaped columellar strut of shorter length may be used primarily to support a short columella caused by inadequate maxillary bone support at its base, or a retracted columella lacking support from either anterior nasal spine or septum.

Wide columella

When the depressor nasi muscles are large the columellar-lip complex is distorted, and the lip may appear to be pulled up into the nose: the columellar-labial angle is wide open and the columellar base wide. Use the skin hook to retract the skin edge and medial crus, and dissect out the bulky muscle. Once identified, clasp the muscle in an artery forceps retracting and dissecting out the deeper portion of the muscle.

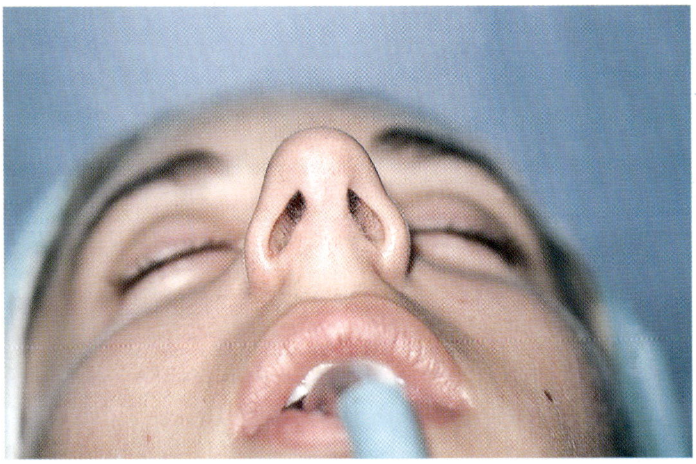

Figure 2.55

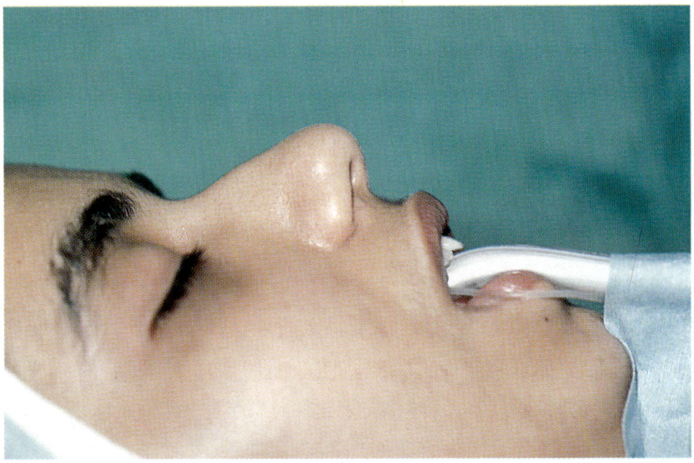

Figure 2.56

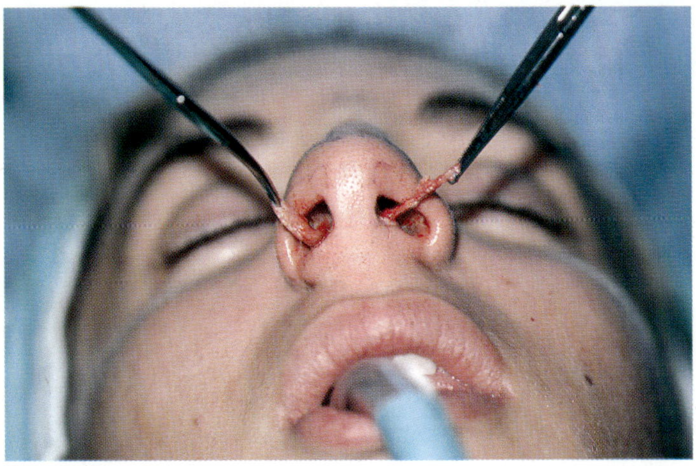

Figure 2.57

Repeat this on the opposite side. At the time of skin closure, use a catgut suture to approximate the medial crura and obliterate the dead space. The posterior end of this suture passes through the anterior border of the septum.

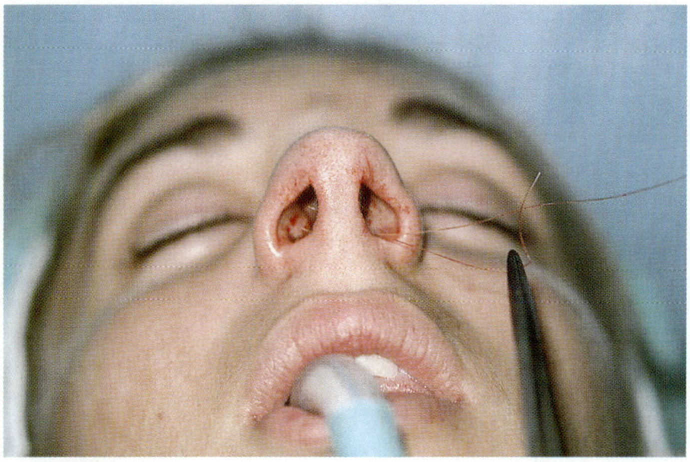

Figure 2.58

Suturing the skin

The first suture of 4.0 catgut establishes the position of the nasal tip.

With the left hand, lightly retract the right nostril margin; at the same time press with the middle finger tip on the supratip. This will approximate the skin edges of the vestibular skin and septum at the correct level. Repeat this on the left side.

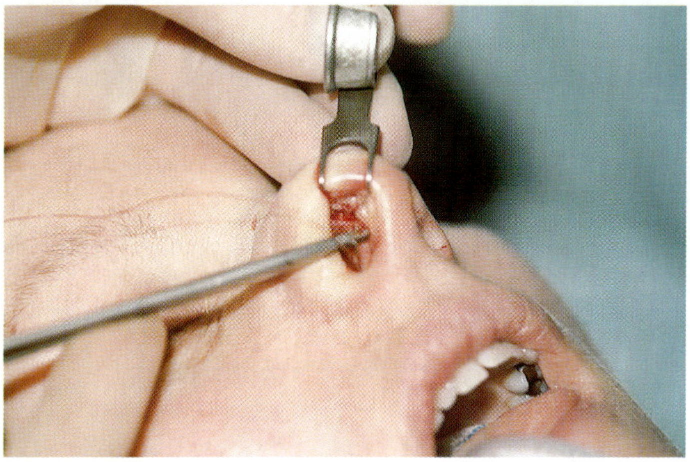

Figure 2.59

Two more sutures approximate the transcartilaginous incision, giving slight eversion to the nostril margin.

Repeat this on the opposite side.

Two more catgut sutures then close the columellar incision on each side.

An additional transfixation suture of 4.0 catgut is used if there is a graft at the columellar base, because this will close off any dead space around the graft. The suture should transfix the septum as it passes posteriorly because this avoids bunching and distortion of the columella when the suture is tightened.

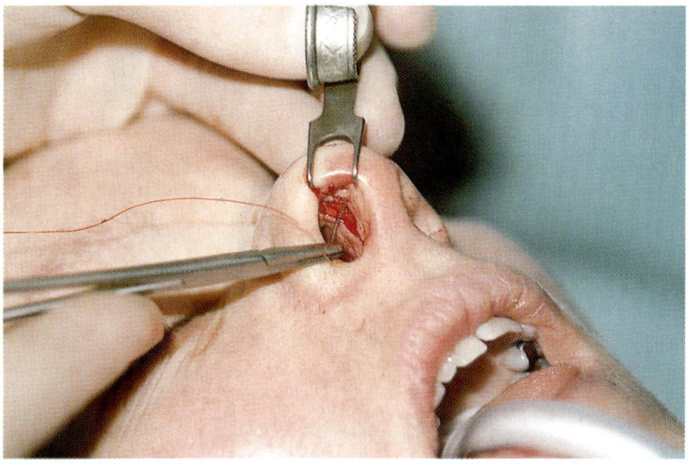

Figure 2.60

Alar base excision

This can occasionally be a part of a basic rhinoplasty, but generally this is a measure reserved for more gross disproportion.

The full extent of nostril flare or excess height of the nostril will only be apparent when the rhinoplasty is complete and the skin incision sutured.

Now examine the alar bases and mark the tissue to be excised.

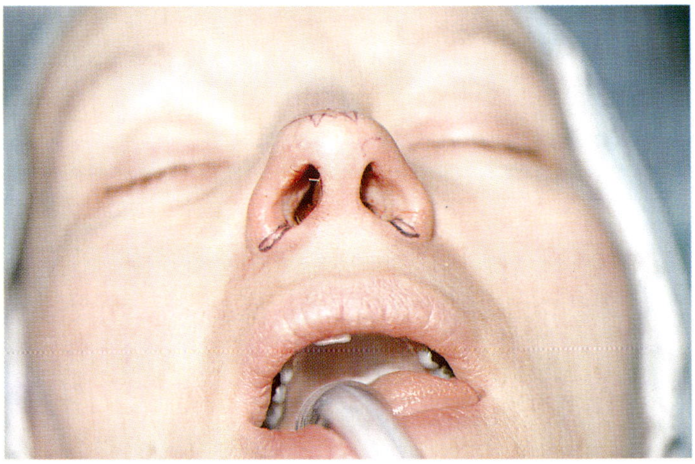

Figure 2.61

To prevent notching at the scar line on the nostril sill, make the incision obliquely, slanting the incisions laterally. Whenever possible minimize the external skin excision where the scar is more conspicuous and the sebaceous skin may heal poorly. Skin closure is with 6.0 nylon.

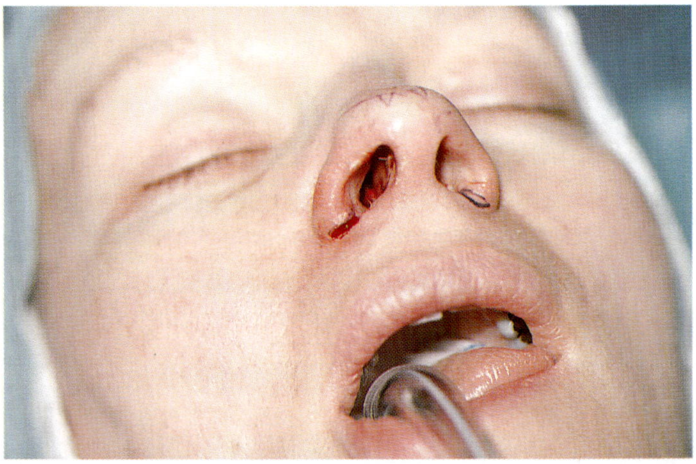

Figure 2.62

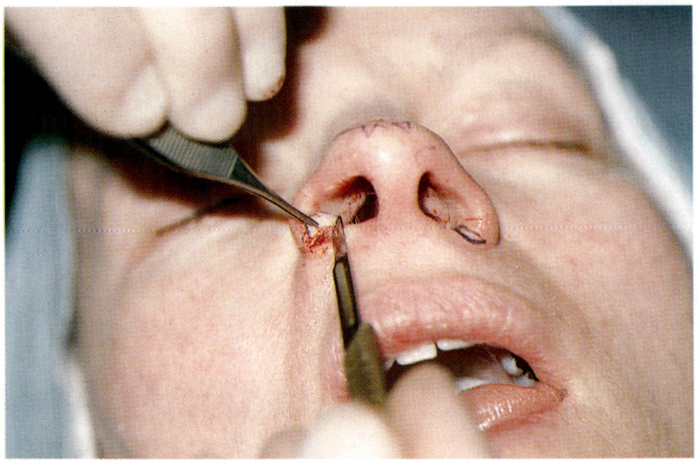

Figure 2.63

For greater detail see page 119.

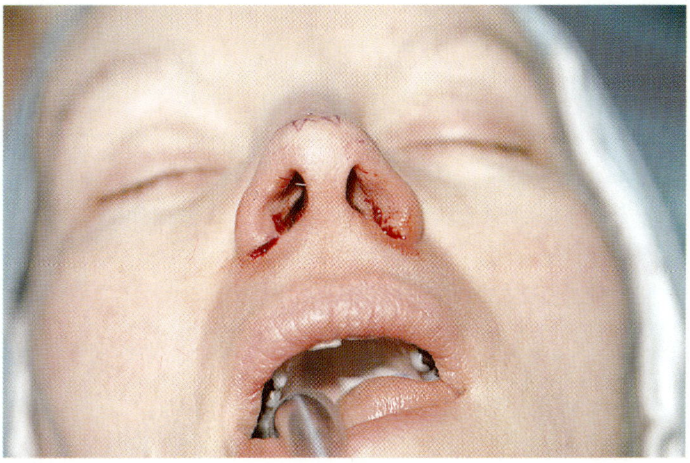

Figure 2.64

Nasal splint and pack

Clear airways

Clean the nostrils with a little hydrogen peroxide and suck out any blood or clot with a no. 12 Jaques catheter. This is important in improving the patient's comfort and airway, and clearing any clot that may remain in the nasopharynx. Do not forget to remove your nasal packs!

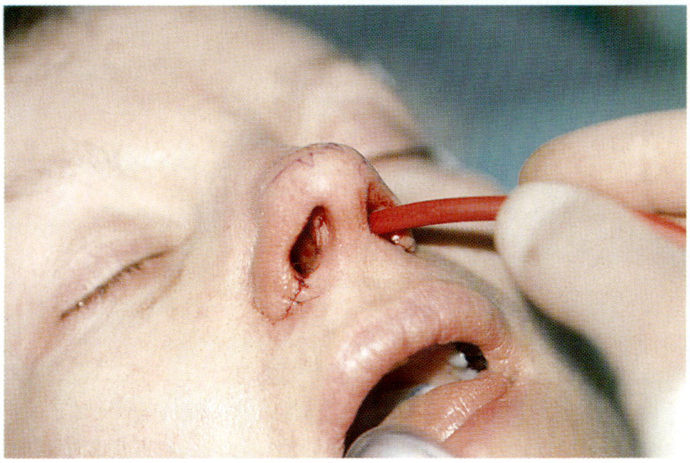

Figure 2.65

Apply 0.25 inch Steristrips to the tip of the nose, then to the dorsum and finally to the glabella, which will help control swelling and adapt the skin to the new nasal skeleton.

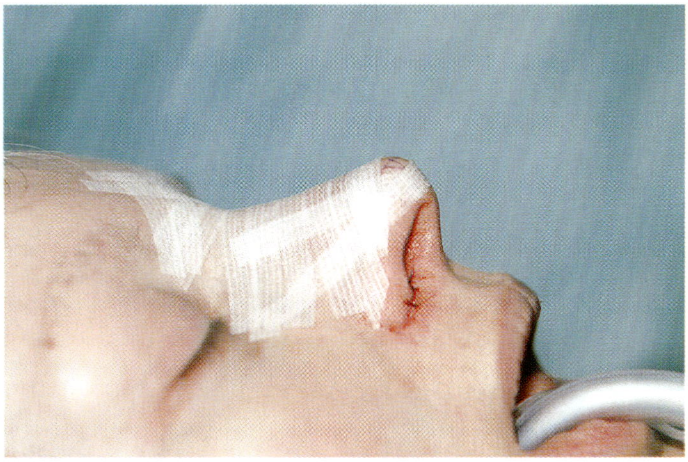

Figure 2.66

Nasal splint

This is cut from a sheet of Orthoplast (Johnson & Johnson) and, after softening in hot water, is dried and cut to size.

Mould and stretch the splint to form the approximate shape, and then apply it while warm to the skin.

Once softened in hot water it is slow to harden and therefore it is unnecessary and dangerous to apply it while hot.

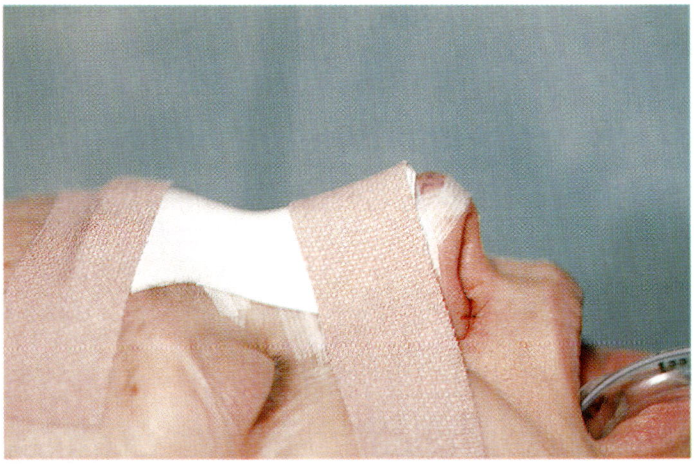

Figure 2.67

Apply ice-cold compresses to harden the splint.

Put a 1 inch wide pink Elastoplast across the cheeks and forehead, compress and secure the splint.

A 4 x 4 inch square of Sofratulle, cut like a trouser pattern and then rolled, makes a convenient nasal pack.

Remove this after 2 hours, clean the nostrils again with hydrogen peroxide and apply antibiotic ointment.

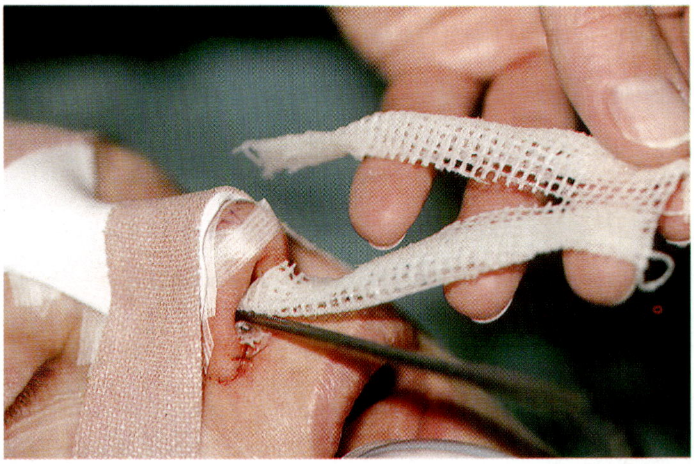

Figure 2.68

Mentoplasty

Introduction

The chin, the nose and forehead are the important features that give balance to the face, especially in the profile view.

Most patients with small chins who seek rhinoplasty are unaware of this feature contributing to their nasal disproportion.

Advising patients in favour of aesthetic surgery is most strongly discouraged, but we have here the one exception. Such advice requires careful supporting analysis and illustrations to inform the patient.

Deformities involving malocclusion, and major malrelationships of mandible and maxilla with associated malocclusion, will not be covered. They are outside the objectives of this book on aesthetic rhinoplasty.

Corrective jaw surgery divides into three main categories:

1. Camouflaging techniques: implants and onlays
2. Osteotomy
3. Contouring.

Most cases of disproportion fall into the category of those only requiring such treatment without interruption of the dentition, and only these will be considered as they are of greatest application to the aesthetic surgeon.

Assessment of the chin

Clinical assessment

A micrognathic jaw will produce a characteristic facial pattern. With the lips relaxed, the lower lip becomes incompetent and, particularly in the lateral view, will appear unsupported, giving a discontented unflattering appearance. With the lips sealed there is an adaptive posture in which the lips and chin may show unattractive strain.

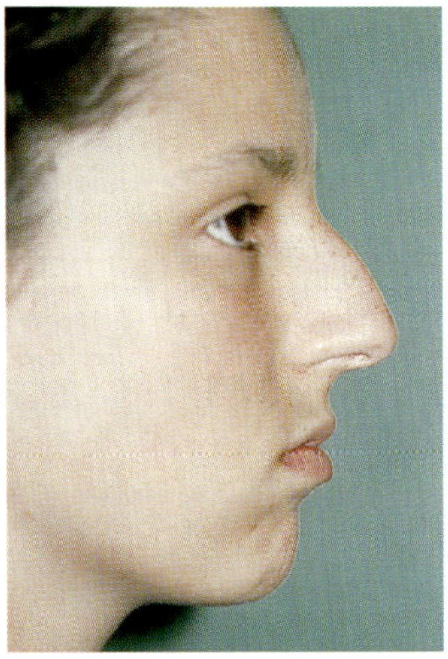

Figure 2.69

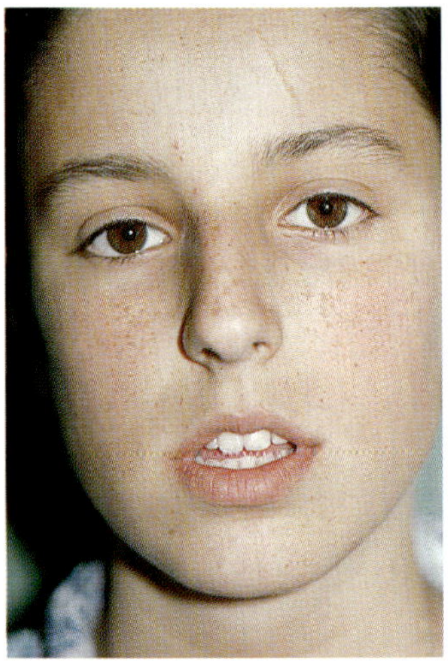

Figure 2.70

Cephalometric analysis

The aesthetic line projected through the nasal tip and upper lip passes near the most anterior bony point of the chin (pogonium). Micrognathia or prognathia lies behind or in front respectively.

Cephalometric radiographs are particularly helpful in visualizing both skeletal framework and soft tissue relationships, although for many simple straightforward cases a lateral radiograph will be sufficient.

Photographs

For guidance of the patient (and relatives) half-plate lateral and full face photographs are invaluable and give a more realistic representation for the patient. A dark background is important and gives a clear facial profile which can then be traced on to paper at the time of consultation. Both the aesthetic line and indicated correction of the chin can be demonstrated and kept as part of the patient's record.

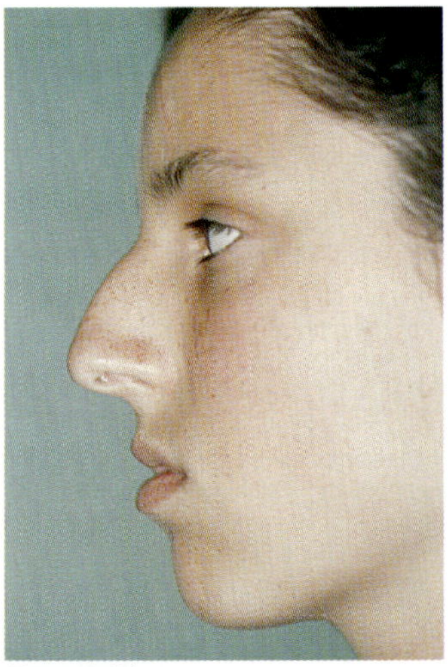

Figure 2.71

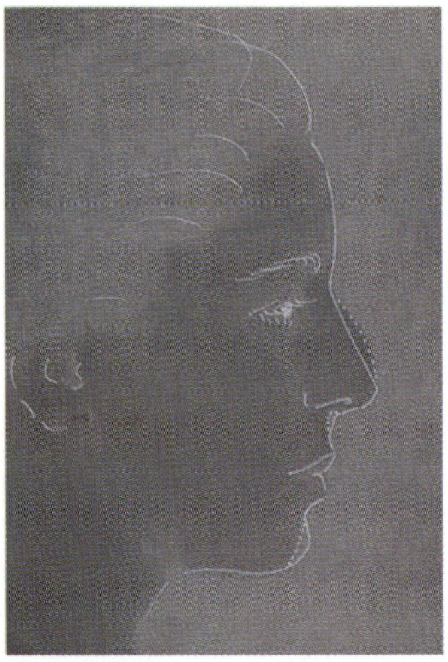

Figure 2.72

Treatment

Camouflaging techniques

Augmentation mentoplasty

Prosthetic augmentation by insertion of a silicone rubber implant, preferably through an intraoral approach, is simple and effective and may be done conveniently under local anaesthetic, although a general anaesthetic may be preferred if combined with rhinoplasty.

A suitable sized implant is selected of which there are many; the longer tapered implants generally give superior results, although a little harder to insert. These newer designs give a more natural appearance and fill out the often narrow angle of the small mandible, where otherwise a shallow depression will be created on either side of the chin. The implant must lie along the edge of the mandible and be precisely positioned centrally to ensure symmetry. Absorption of the underlying bone can occur, especially if the implant is wrongly placed over the softer alveolar bone, or inaccurately fitted against the underlying bony surface.

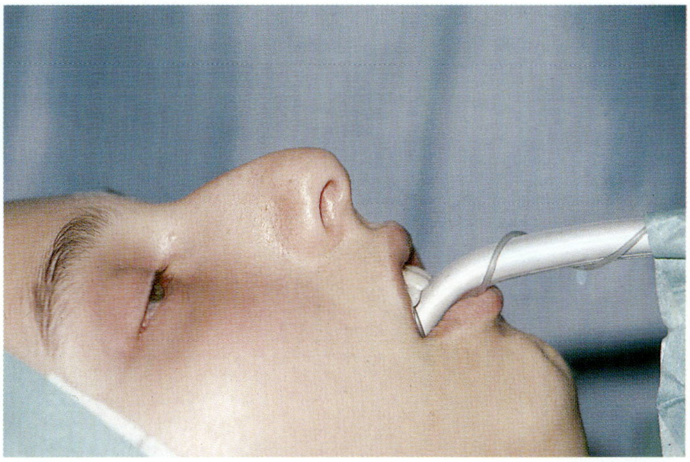

Figure 2.73

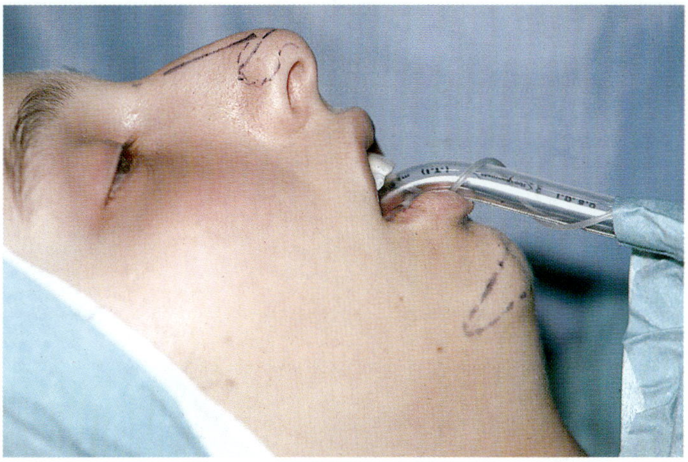

Figure 2.74

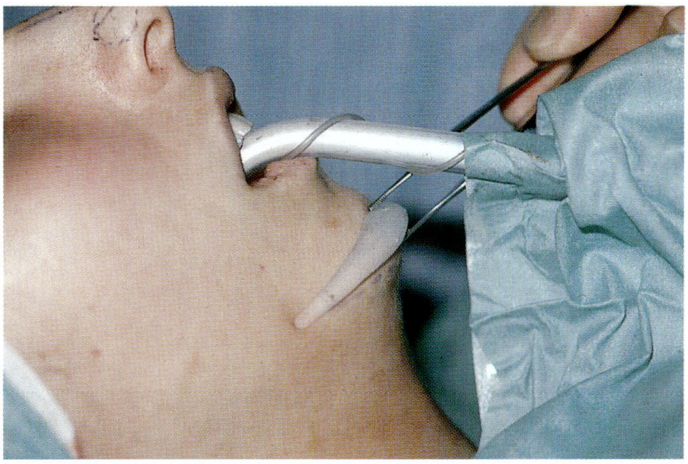

Figure 2.75

Technique

1. The size and position of the implant is marked on the skin, and the soft tissues infiltrated with 0.5% lignocane and adrenaline 1:200 000.

2. The mucosal incision will vary depending on the size of the implant. Usually a 3 cm incision is sufficient, and is made a few millimetres superior to the labial sulcus to ensure sufficient mucosal free edge for easy suturing.

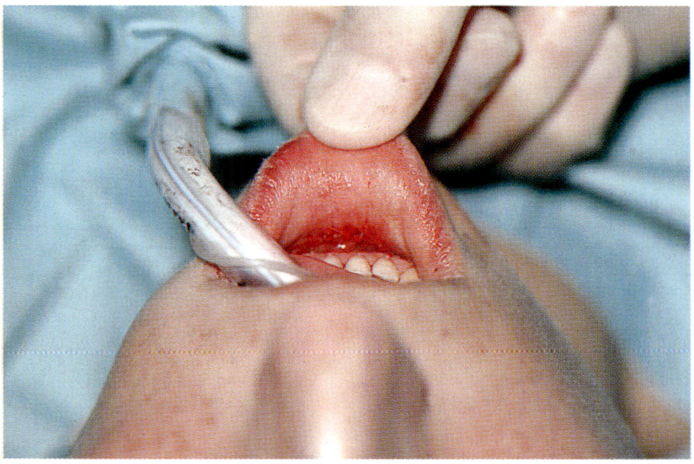

Figure 2.76

3. Open the mid-line space between the paired mentalis muscles by sharp dissection down to the mandibular bone.

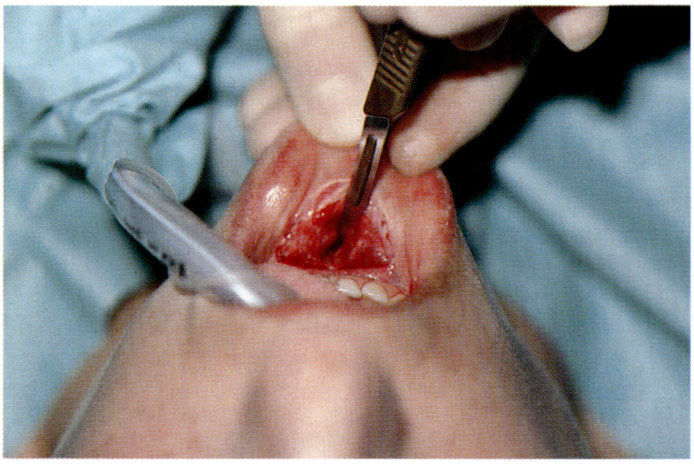

Figure 2.77

4. Use a periosteal elevator to extend the space subperiosteally down to the inferior margin of the mandible, and then laterally along the same plane. The Terino elevator is excellent for this purpose.

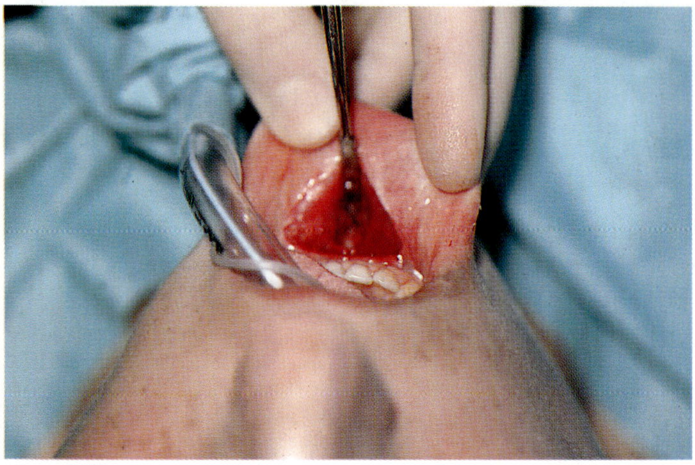

Figure 2.78

5. Using scissors gently stretch up the inelastic periosteum and muscle to make sufficient space for the implant. Carefully avoid damage to the mental nerve as it exits through the mental foramen.

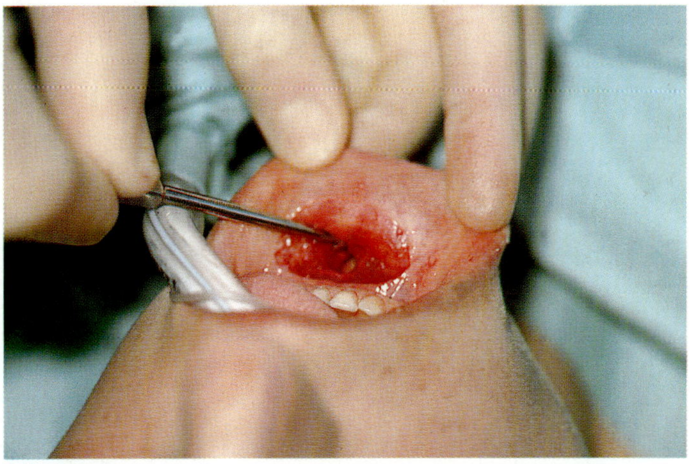

Figure 2.79

6. Insert the implant tightly folded and held with the thumb and forefinger. 'Feed' the lateral ends of the implant into the side pockets by a combination of gentle pressure and sliding of the ends of the implant. If the pocket is too tight it will need to be further enlarged and the manoeuvre repeated.

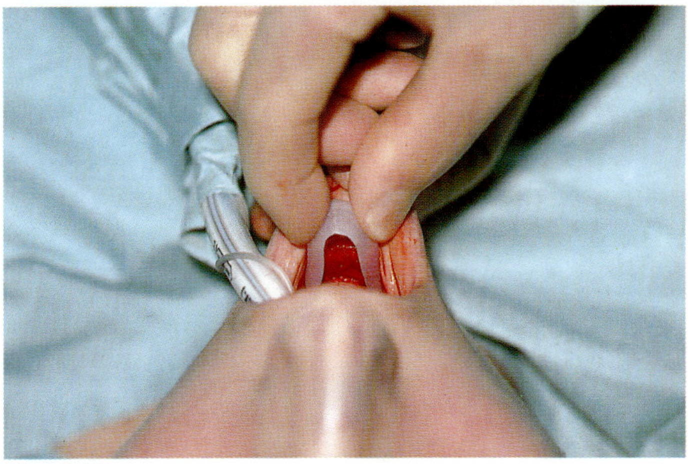

Figure 2.80

7. Gently probe the lateral pockets with the osteotome to check that the implant is not folded on itself, and that it lies centrally. Most implants have a central marking line or perforation.

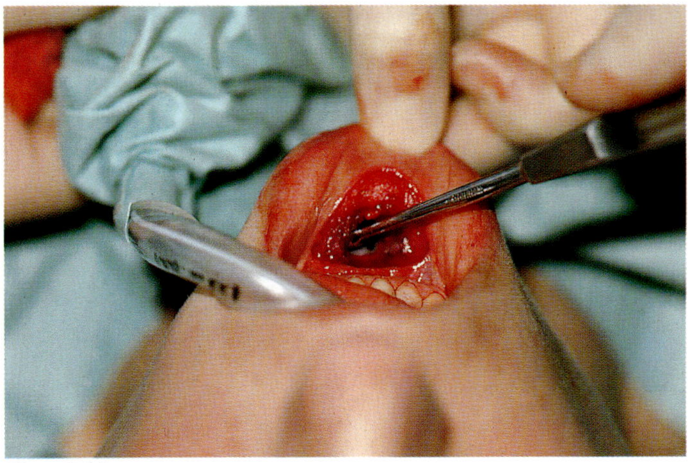

Figure 2.81

Secure the implant in the mid-line with a 4.0 catgut suture through the central hole and overlying muscle.

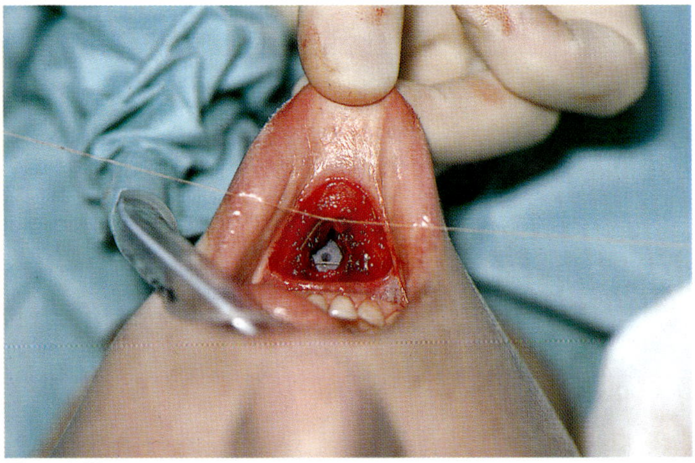

Figure 2.82

8. Close the mentalis muscle first with two interrupted 4.0 catgut sutures.

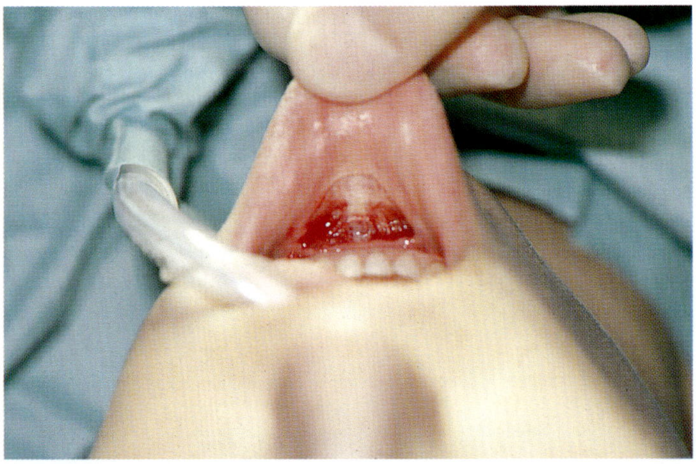

Figure 2.83

9. Close the mucous membrane with a running 4.0 catgut suture. Preservation of a cuff of mucous membrane on the gingival side makes this closure much easier.

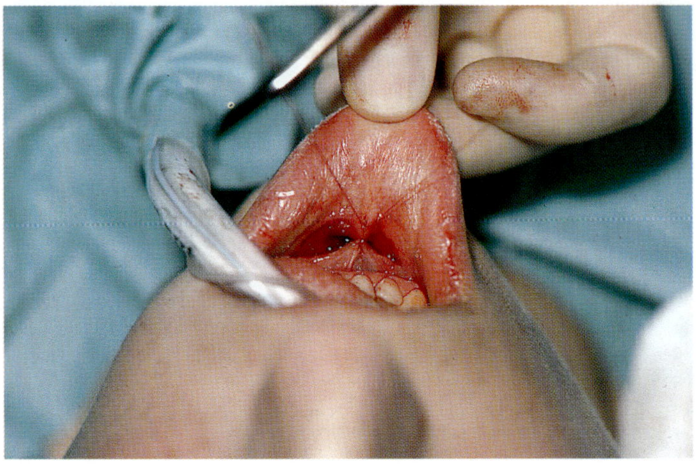

Figure 2.84

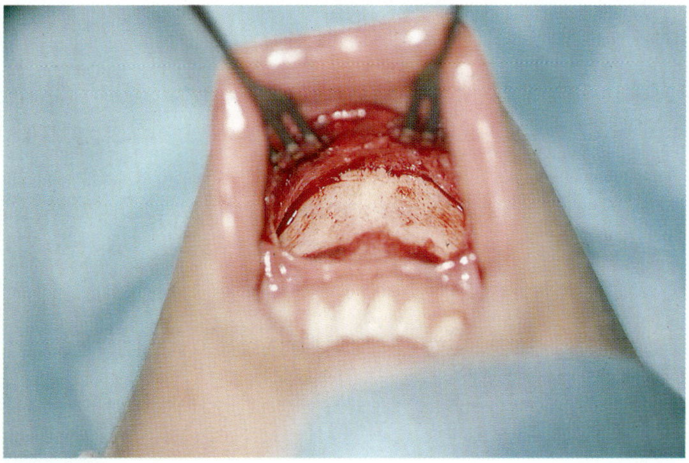

Figure 2.85

Pre- and postoperative examples of combined rhinoplasty and chin augmentation.

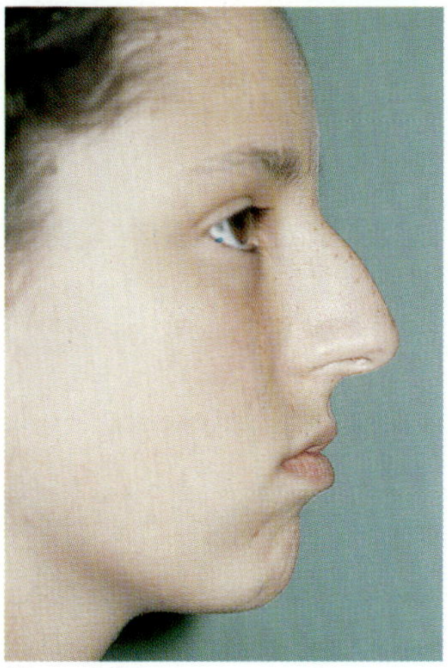

Figure 2.86

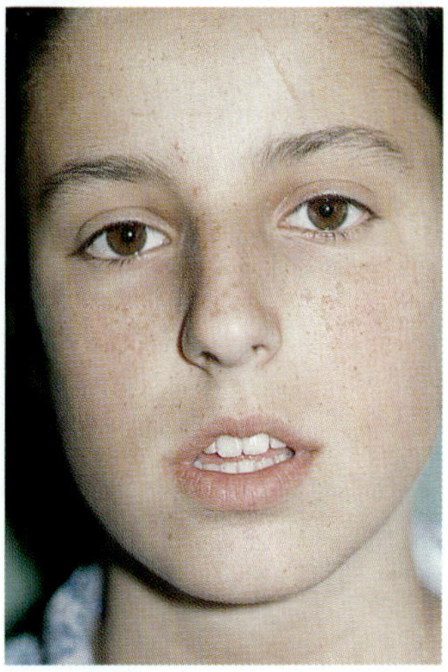

Figure 2.87

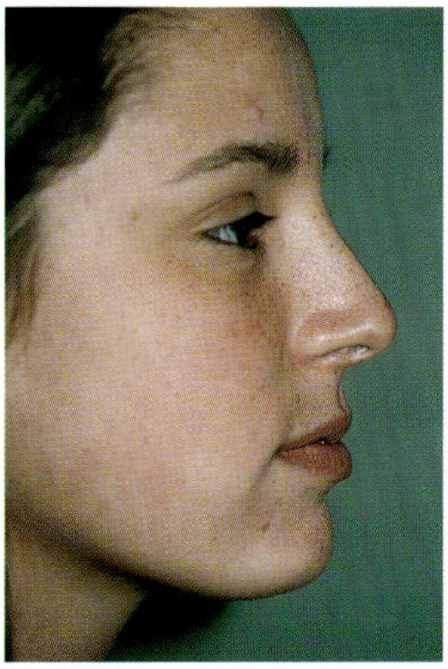

Figure 2.88

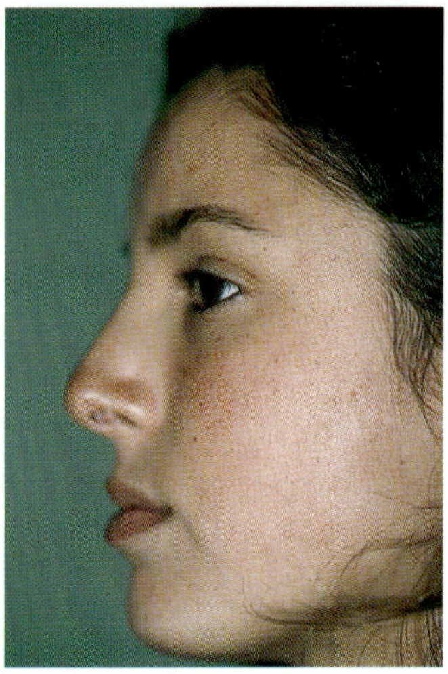

Figure 2.89

Osteotomy

Horizontal osteotomy

The micrognathic chin can be brought forward surgically by sectioning of the mandible in a horizontal or oblique plane inferior to the mental nerve. This is especially suitable for solving problems where there is increased vertical height or asymmetry. Obviously the exact optimum line of the osteotomy must be calculated beforehand with the use of radiograph and photographs as previously discussed.

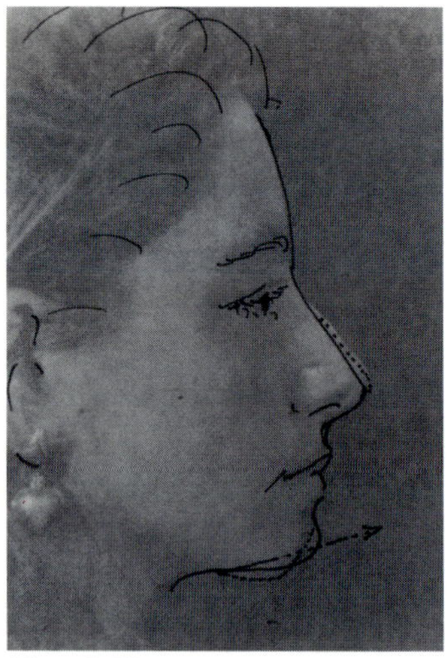

Figure 2.90

A more extensive intraoral operation is involved than in augmentation mentoplasty. The muscles are left attached to the bone fragment to be advanced and fixed internally. Wedge resection of the bone may be performed at the same time and is the ideal operation for such cases where there is excess vertical height or asymmetry.

Technique

1. Make the mucosal incision on the labial side of the lower sulcus out to the level of the second premolar tooth on each side.
2. Strip the soft tissues and periosteum off the anterior mandible, carefully exposing the mental nerve and its exit point at the foramen, opposite the first premolar tooth.
3. Mark the proposed line of osteotomy ensuring that this runs obliquely on to the inferior margin of the bone, avoiding a palpable angle. Make a mid-line marking with the saw to ensure accurate reapproximation following bone resection.
4. Perform the osteotomy, ensuring water irrigation to cool the bone, and direct observation and preservation of both mental nerves.
5. To gain further forward mobilization of the bone fragment, gently lever open the line of osteotomy, thereby stretching up the periosteal attachment along its inner margin.

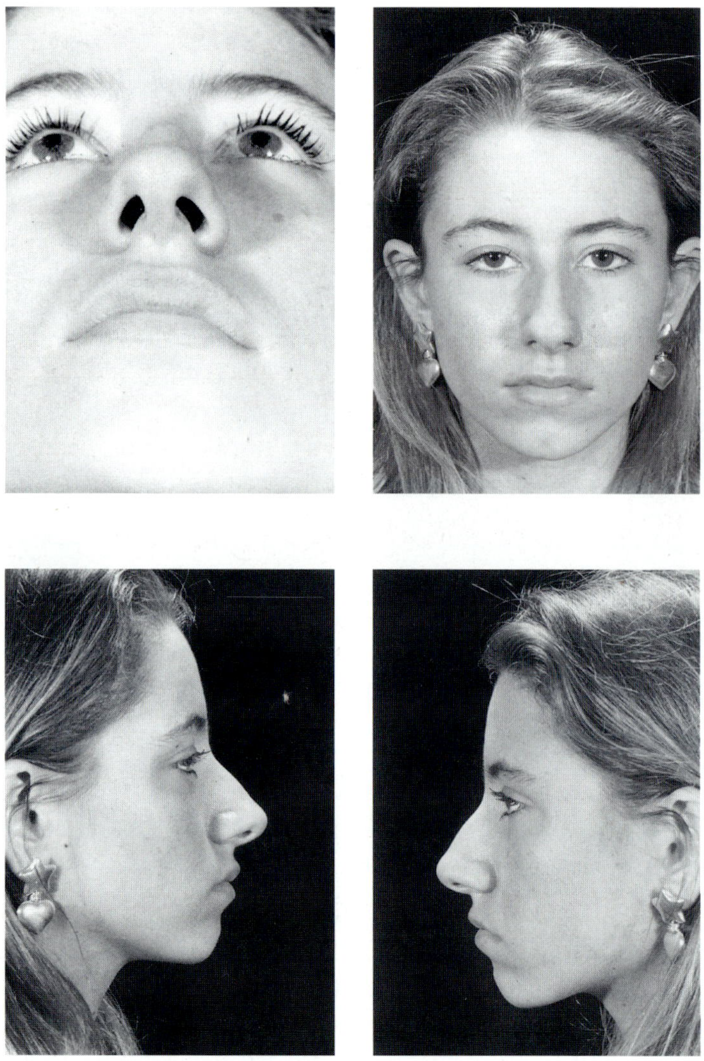

6. Draw the bony fragment forward (with muscles attached) to the desired point, and secure by two Kirschner wires. These wires must be angled in a direction that prevents separation of the osteotomy, as well as maintaining forward position of the anterior bone fragment.
7. Cut the Kirschner wires off flush with the bone.
8. Irrigate the wound clean of all bone dust and fragments.

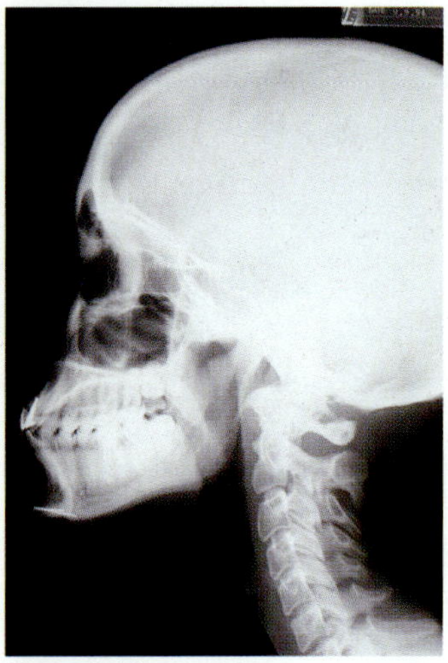

Figure 2.91

Palpate the inferior mandibular margin to ensure that this is free of any palpable 'step'. Smooth off with a rasp if necessary.

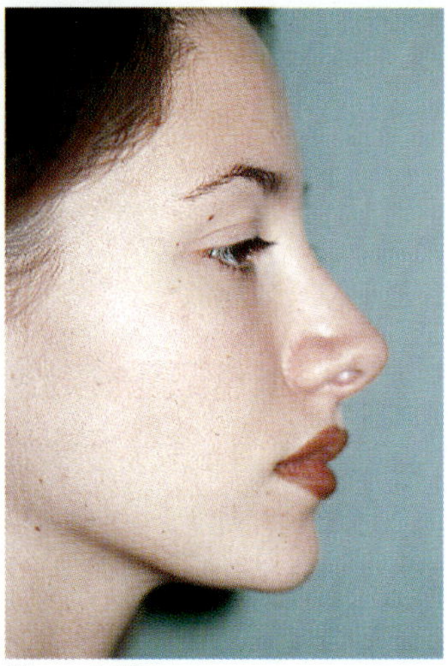

Figure 2.92

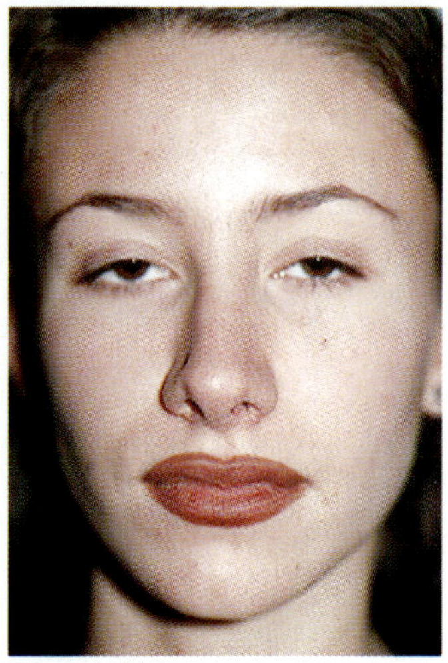

Figure 2.93

Close the muscle and mucosa as already described for augmentation mentoplasty.
Following surgery apply a light pressure dressing, and continue antibiotics and mouth washes for a week. Maintain graduated soft diet for 3 weeks, and avoid any excessive stress to the mandible for 5 weeks.

Fixation plates may also provide a solid and precise option.

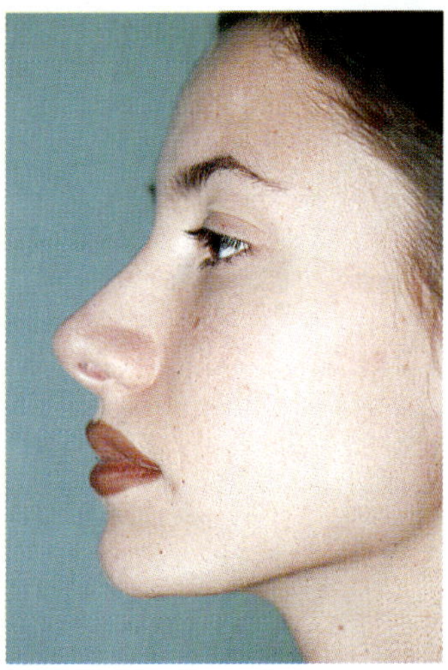

Figure 2.94

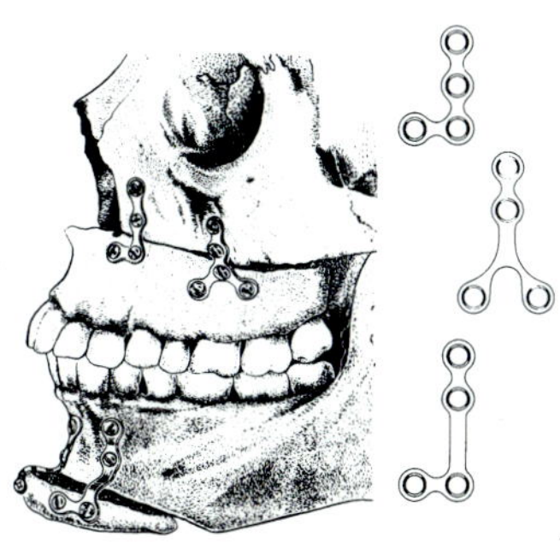

Figure 2.95

Wedge osteotomy

This is an ideal solution for cases where there is also excess vertical height or asymmetry. Again a careful analysis is made preoperatively.

Technique

Follow the same steps as for the previously described horizontal or oblique osteotomy, but remove a suitable wedge of mandible after completing the initial bone separation.

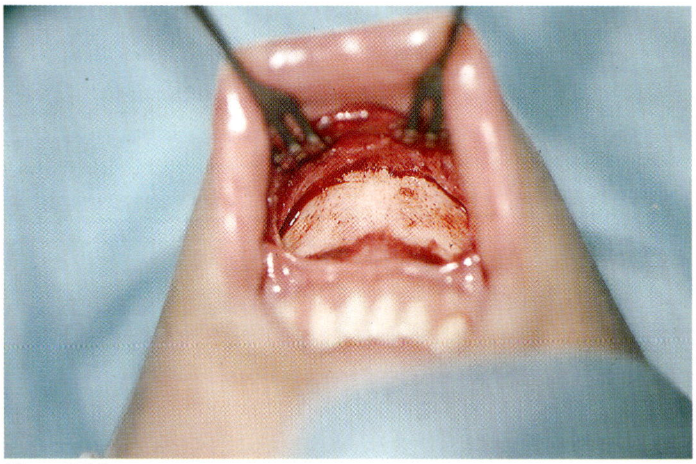

Figure 2.96

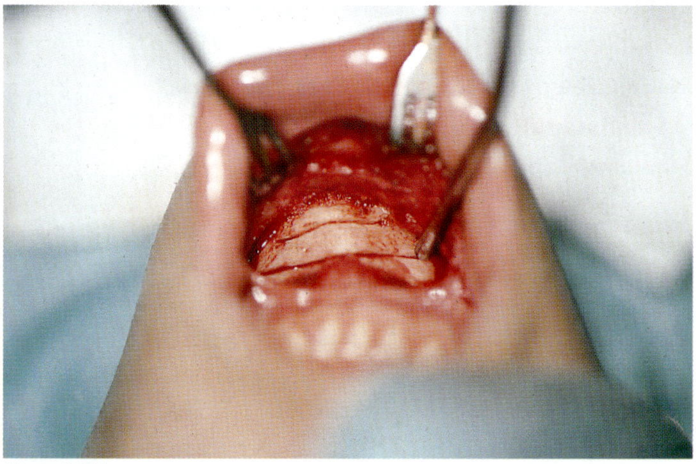

Figure 2.97

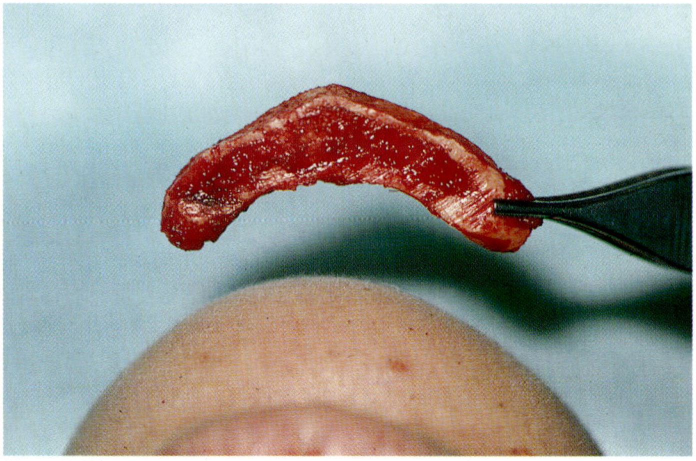

Figure 2.98

Two Kirschner wires are inserted for fixation and cut off flesh with the bone surface.

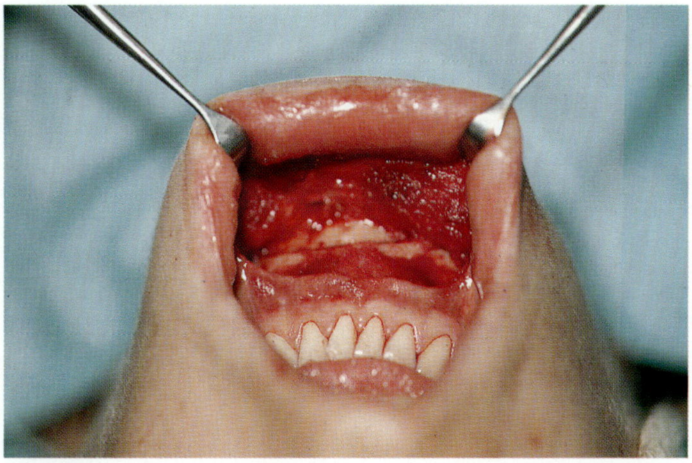

Figure 2.99

Clinical example of wedge osteotomy
Preoperative views

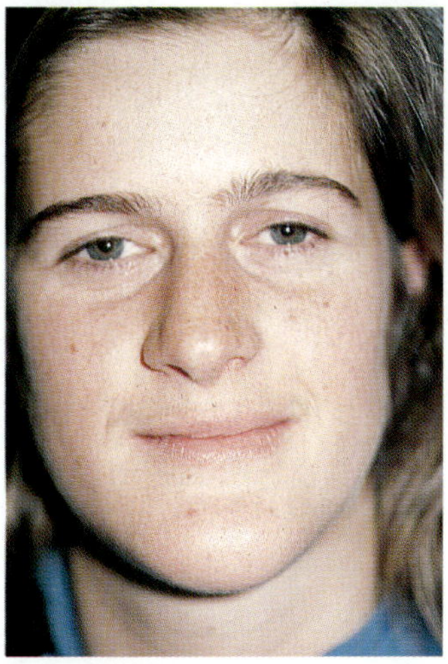

Figure 2.100a

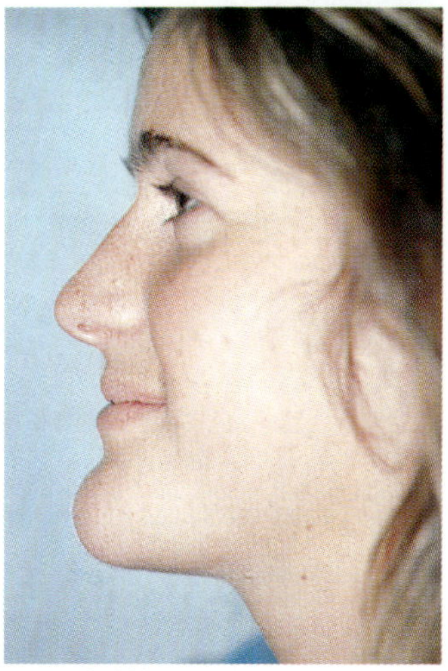

Figure 2.100c

One year after the operation

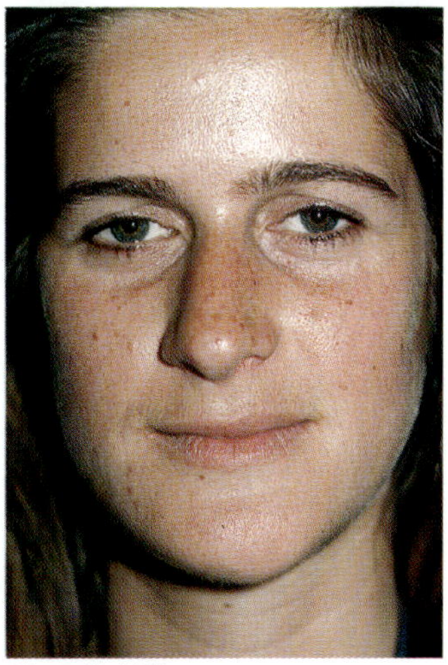

Figure 2.100b

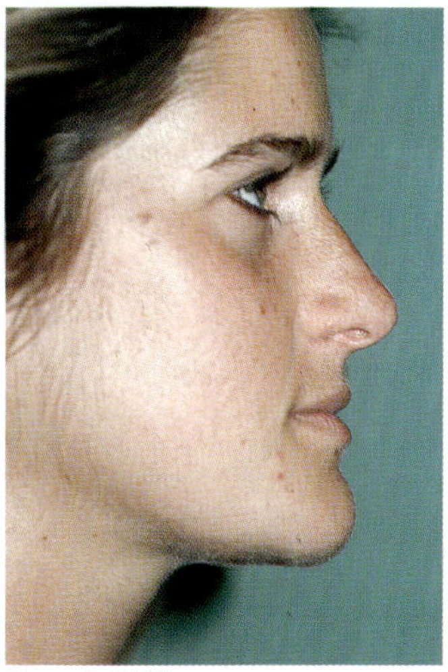

Figure 2.100d

Mandibular contouring

There are certain cases where minor prominence of the chin profile can be reduced by simple and direct excision of bone. This is done only for cases of anterior prominence not greater than 4 mm. All cases greater than this and all cases where the excess prominence lies in an inferior direction should be treated by wedge excision or sliding osteotomy.

The following is an example of minor anterior reduction mentoplasty by direct excision.

The technique follows the same steps for bone exposure, and the bone is then reduced and suitably contoured by a bone cutting burr and saw if necessary.

Conclusion

The aesthetic surgeon is well advised to consult and cooperate with a maxillofacial surgeon in all cases of a grosser or more complex nature, where more extensive analysis or assessment of the dental occlusion should be carried out.

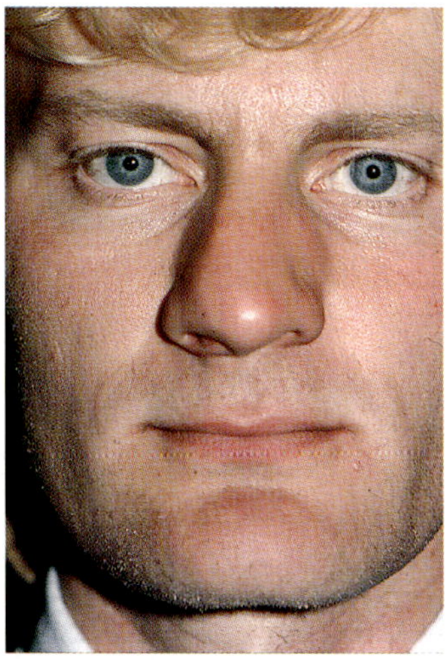

Figure 2.101a

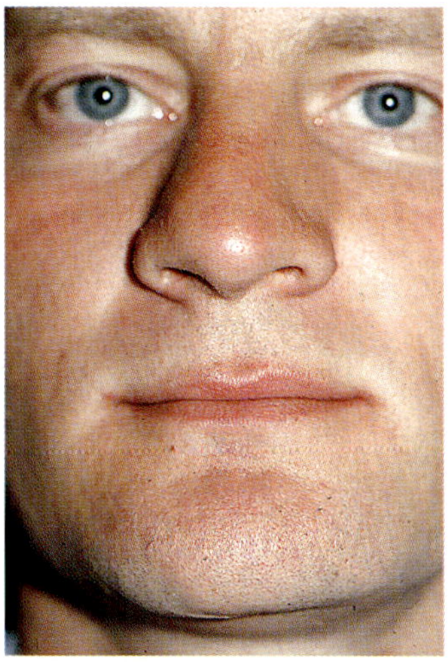

Figure 2.102a

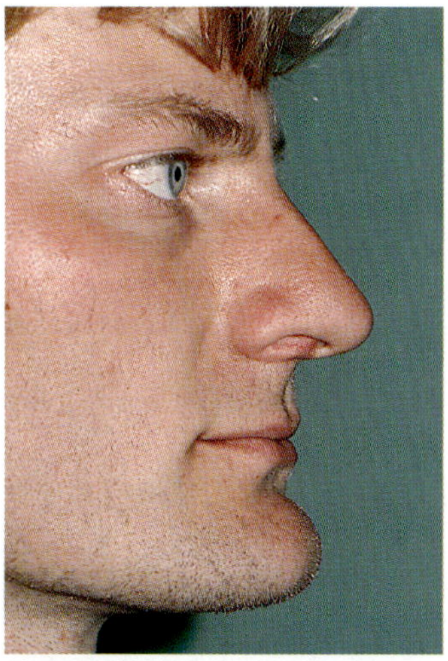

Figure 2.101b

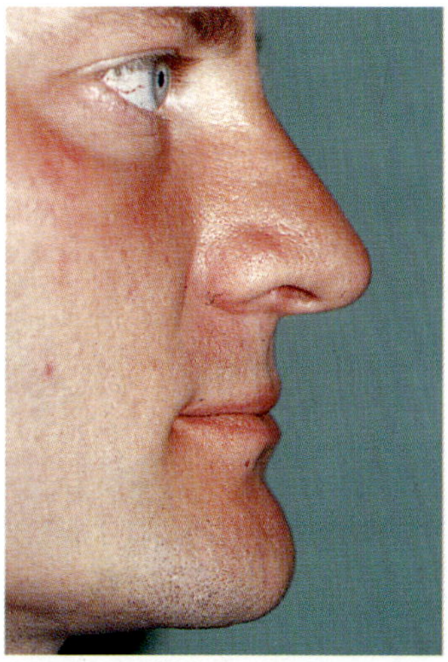

Figure 2.102b

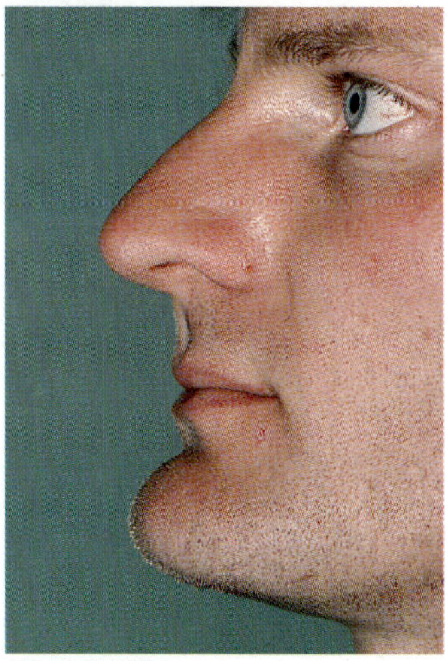

Figure 2.101c

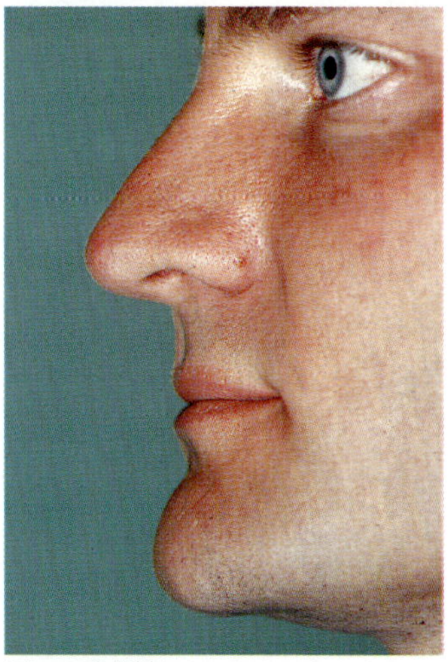

Figure 2.102c

Preoperative

One year postoperative

Part III

ADJUNCTIVE TECHNIQUES

Tip

Broad tip

The basic rhinoplasty technique already described gives slight narrowing and refinement of the tip by excision of the excess cephalic portion of the lateral crura (page 17).

A moderately wide tip will require wedge excision as described below. This narrows the tip but also approximates the cephalic edges of the lateral crura, which in turn give slight eversion or flare to the nostril margins. The effect is aesthetically pleasing.

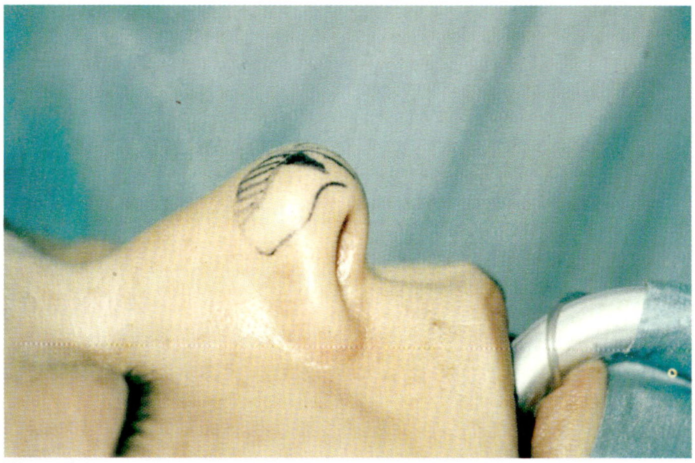

Figure 3.1

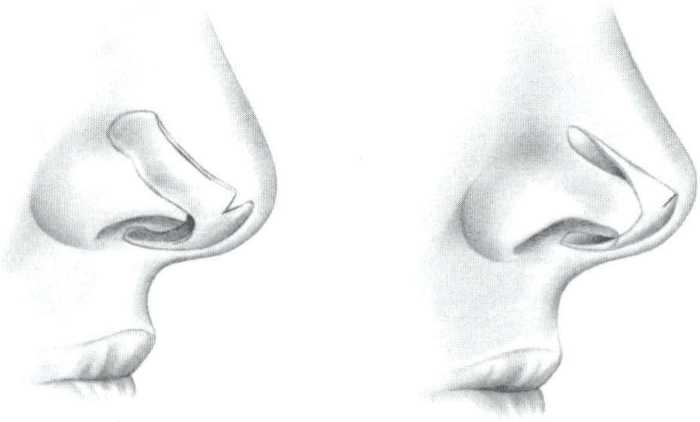

Figure 3.2

Mark the apex of the nasal vault by light pressure with a no. 15 scalpel.

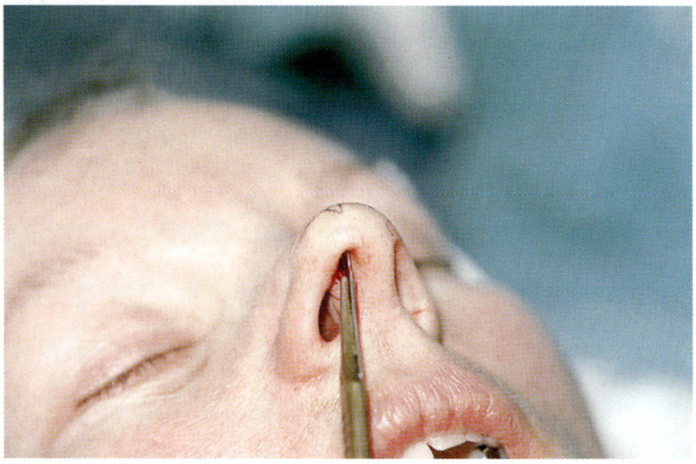

Figure 3.3

Complete this incision under direct vision, and remove a wedge on the lateral side. This incision does not extend through more than 50% of the width of the cartilage.

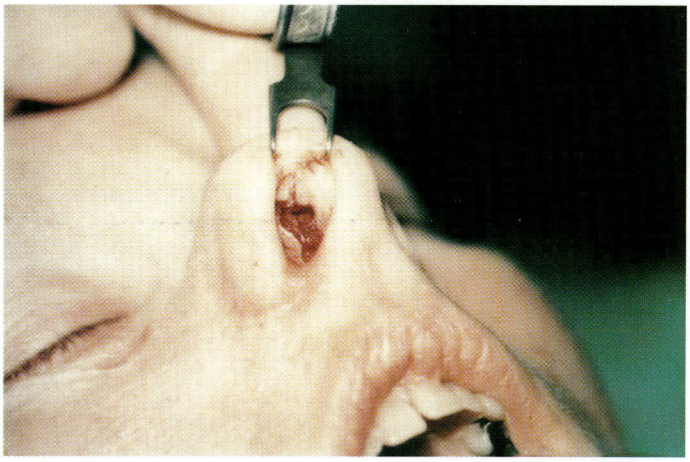

Figure 3.4

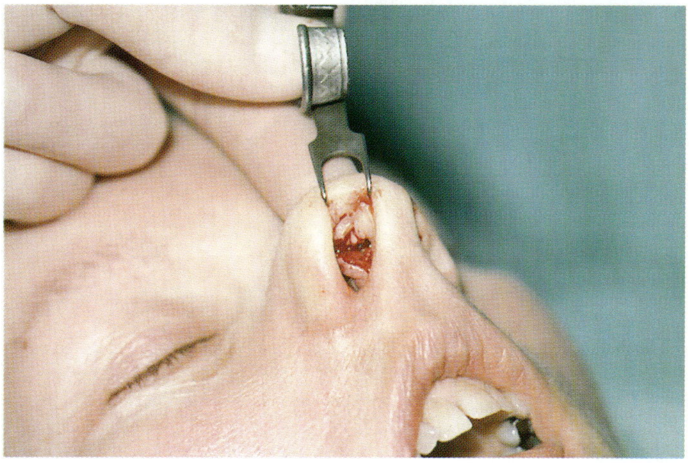

Figure 3.5

Repeat this procedure on the left side.

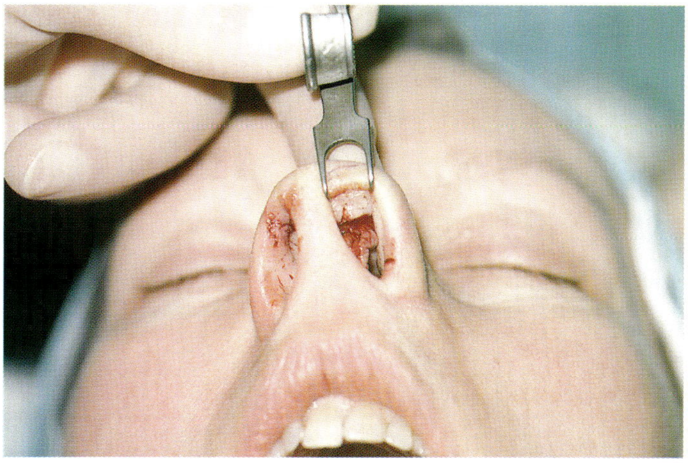

Figure 3.6

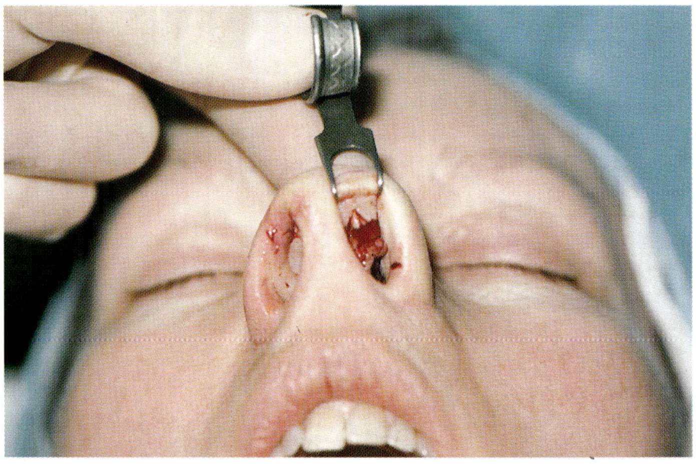
Figure 3.7

The tip is blunt and round before any cartilage excision.

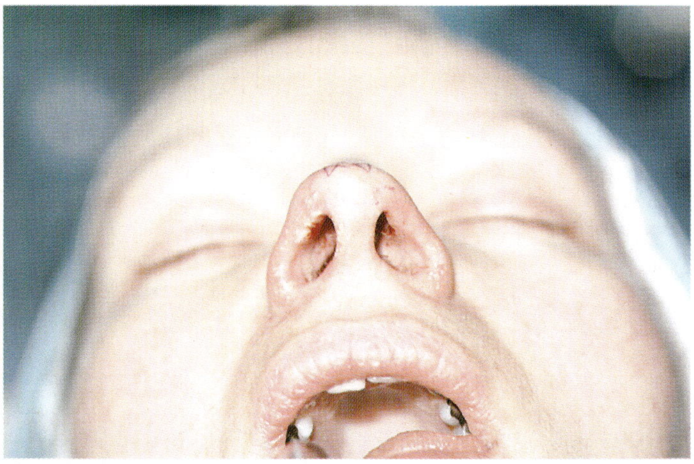
Figure 3.8

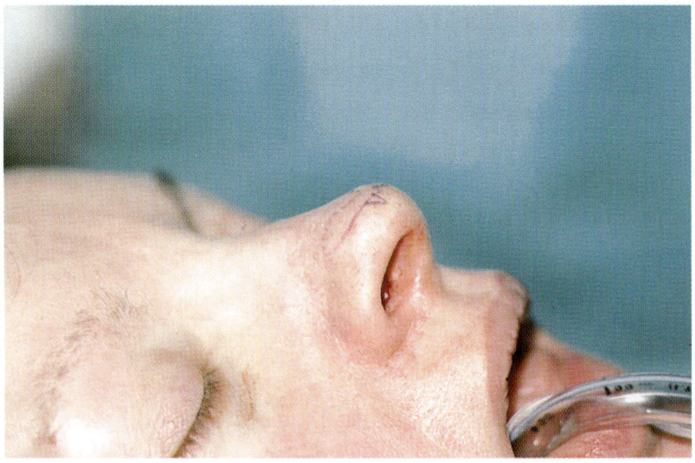
Figure 3.9

The tip is narrowed after simple removal of the cephalic portion of the tip cartilage.

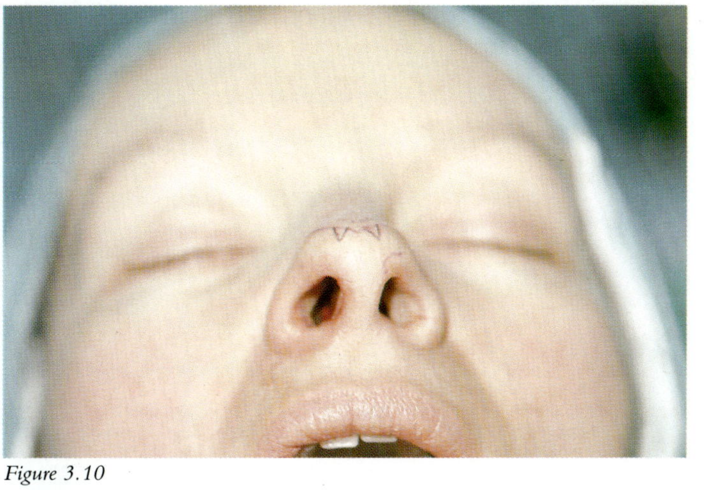

Figure 3.10

A more angular and subtle tip definition results from conservative wedge excision. Never carry this through more than 50% of the width of the tip cartilage without also applying an onlay graft, otherwise an ugly knuckle will eventually develop.
The wedge excision is closed with 4.0 catgut at the same time as the other internal nasal incisions.

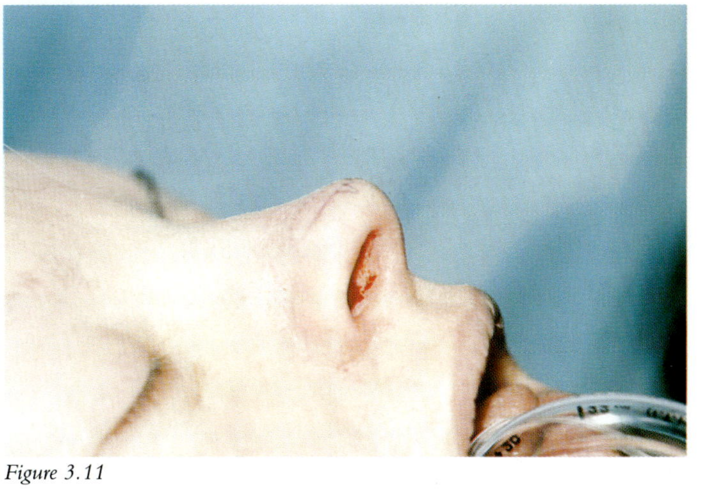

Figure 3.11

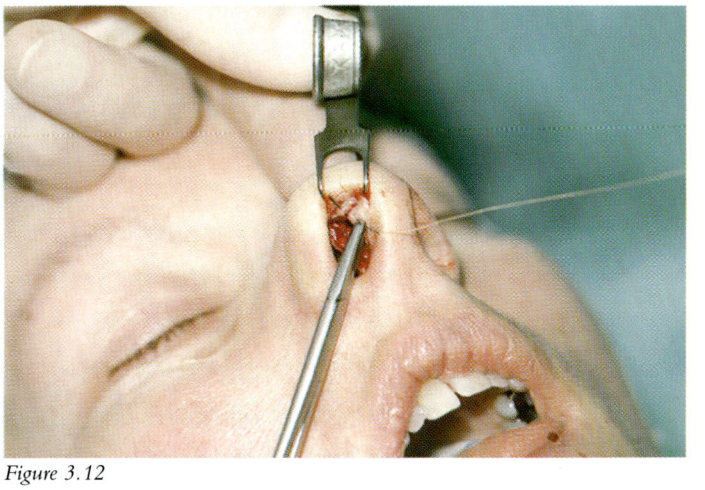

Figure 3.12

For more major reduction of the nasal tip, segmental resection of the dome and an onlay tip graft gives a reliable long-term result.

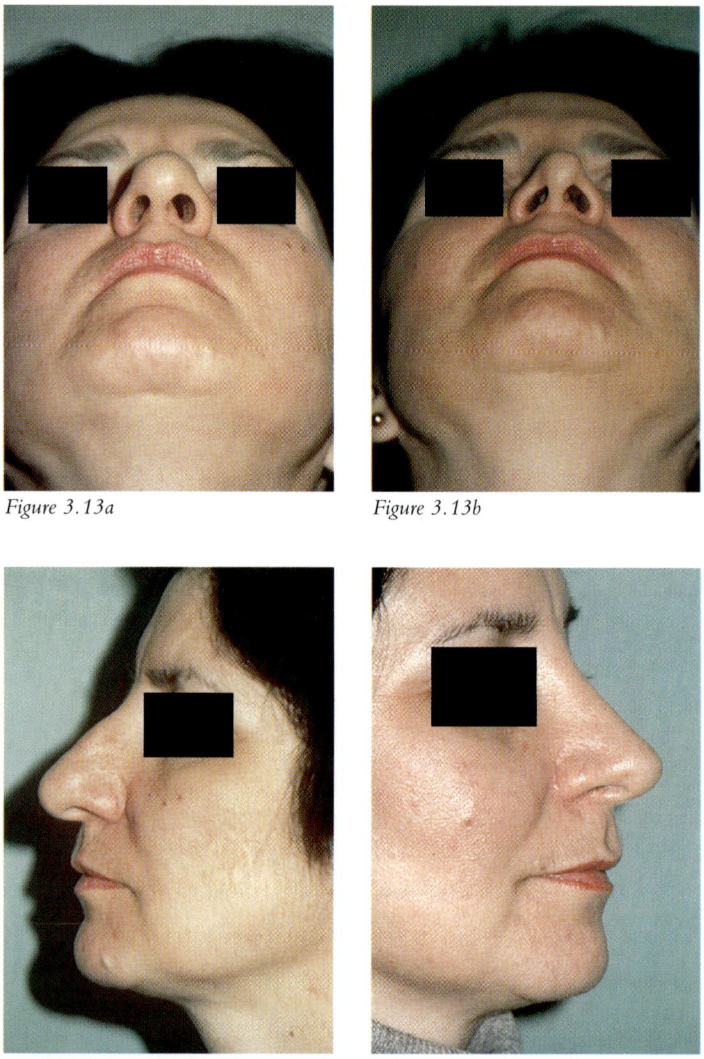

Figure 3.13a

Figure 3.13b

Figure 3.13c

Figure 3.13d

High tip

The basic rhinoplasty already described can lower the tip slightly both by reduction of the lateral crura and by release of soft tissue attachment at the base of the columella.

A high tip may be caused by a disproportionately long or large columella, or prominence of the vestibular portion of the tip cartilages.

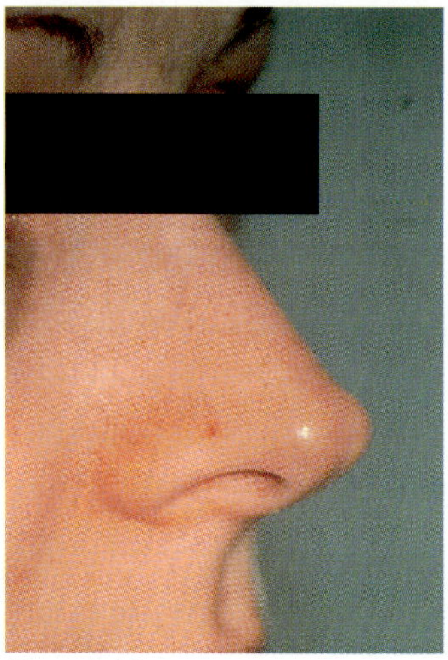

Figure 3.14

A high nasal tip caused primarily by excess prominence of the vestibular cartilage will need reduction of this cartilage.
The dome of the tip cartilage is exposed through a rim incision.
The cartilage is separated from the skin with fine dissecting scissors.
The cartilages are then 'bucket handled' forward.

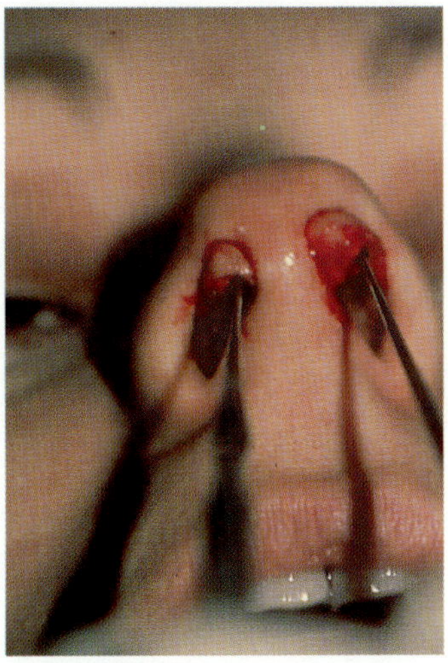
Figure 3.15

The cut edges of cartilage are approximated with two 6.0 nylon sutures. The cartilage is overlapped to ensure firmer fixation.

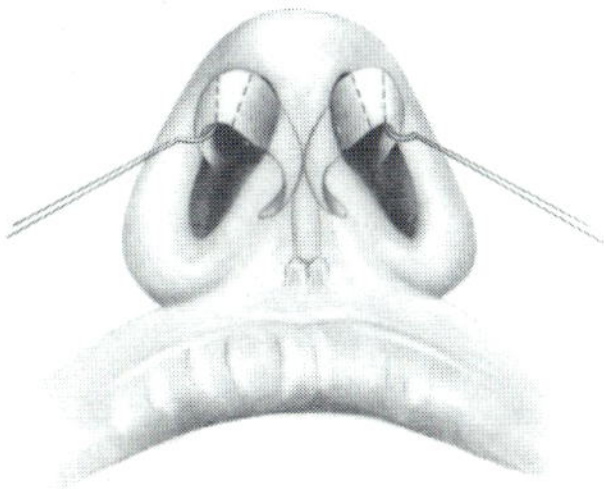
Figure 3.16

The desired width of cartilage is excised as a wedge, preserving the nasal lining.
An onlay graft of bilobular shape is inserted over the two domes to ensure pleasing definition of the tip, and an abutment for the cut ends of the tip cartilage.

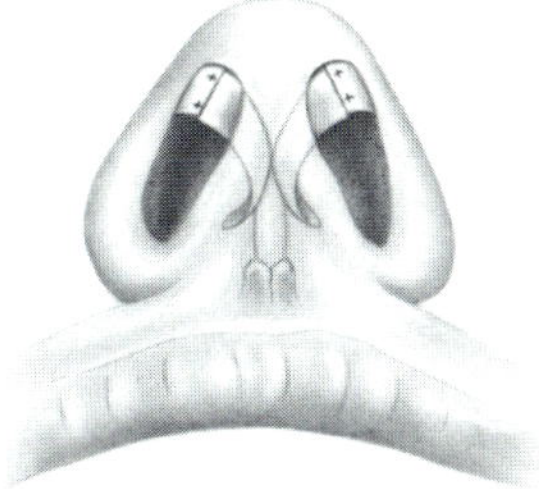
Figure 3.17

Precise fixation with a suture is necessary because there is obviously no soft tissue pocket surrounding and stabilizing the graft in position.

The incision is closed with 6.0 catgut sutures. Other techniques, such as scoring the cartilaginous domes, the Lipsett manoeuvre or excision of three small cartilaginous triangles (Millard), can achieve the same reduction, but in my hands do not create a tip definition that is pleasing.

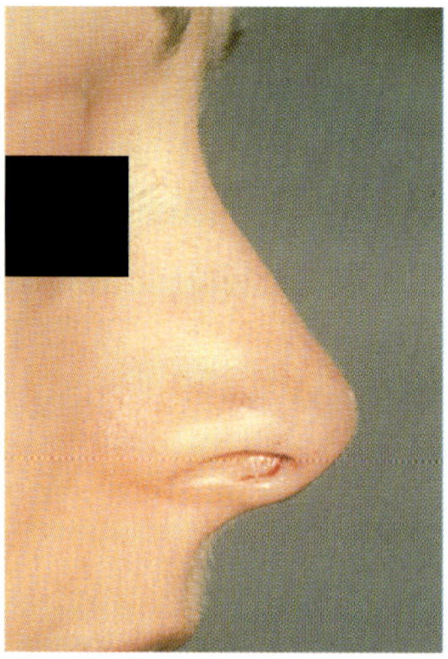

Figure 3.18a

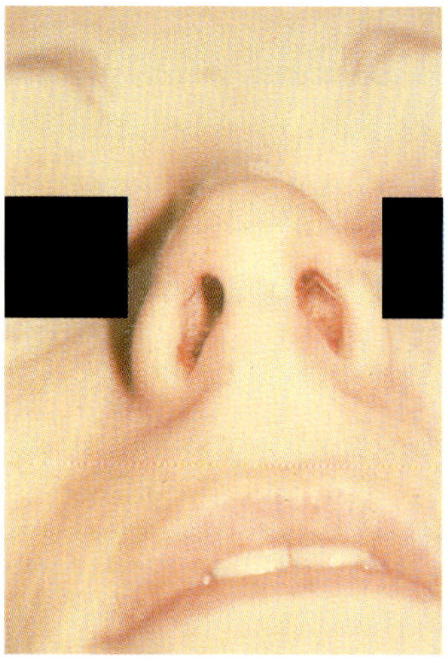

Figure 3.18b

To shorten the columella, dissect out the base of the medial crus; this is very closely attached to the skin, so care must be taken.

Excise a 3 mm length which is usually appropriate. Repeat this on the opposite side.

This manoeuvre is similar to shortening the base of a tent pole. The nasal tip will drop and the columellar soft tissues adapt to a slightly shortened length.

If after suturing the columella there is excess skin at the base, this small ridge is excised.

Do not extend this wedge too anteriorly as it will then cause an unattractive sharp columellar-labial angle when approximated by sutures.

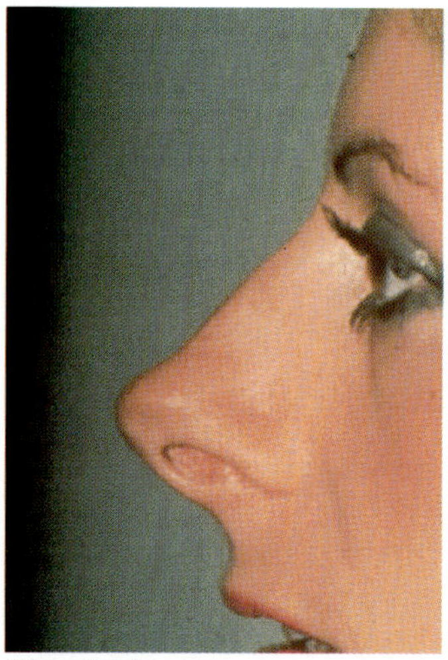

Figure 3.19a

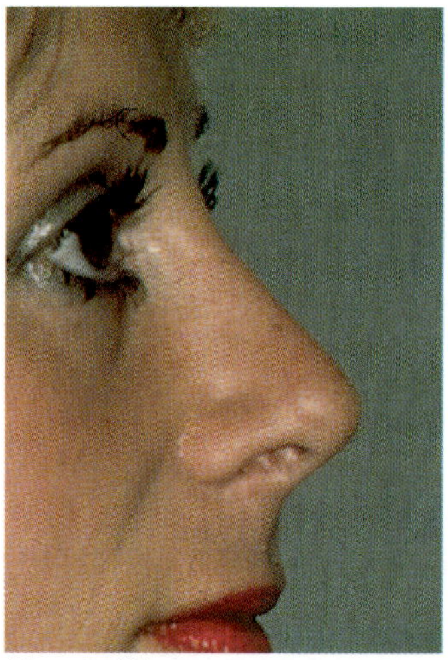

Figure 3.19b

Bulbous tip

In contrast to the broad tip which is more apparent in the frontal view, the bulbous tip is more conspicuous in the lateral view. This is caused by the high rounded contour of the cephalic portion of the lateral crus, which forms the highest point of the tip profile.

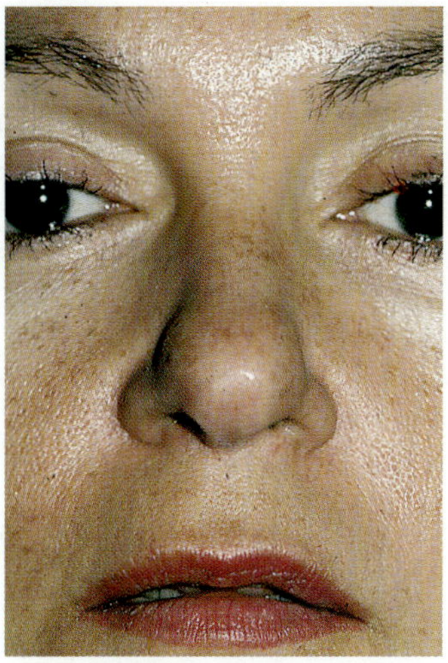

Figure 3.20

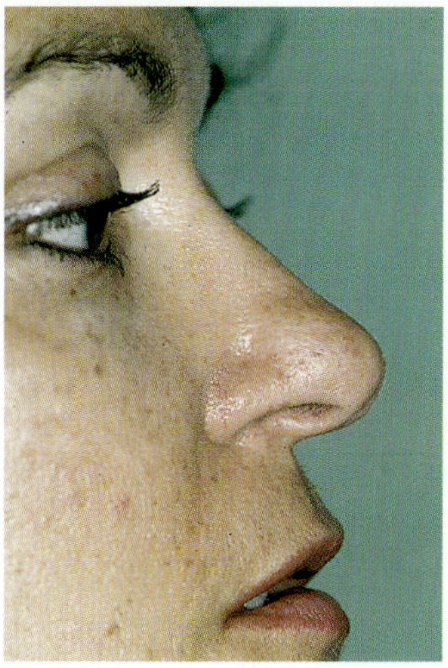

Figure 3.21

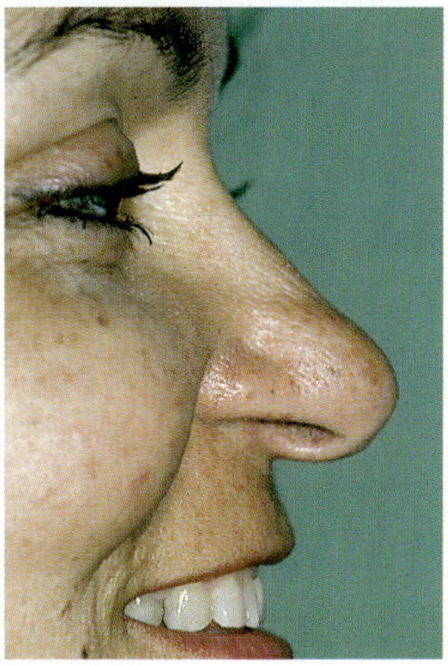

Figure 3.22

Remove the cephalic portion of the lateral crus.

Convert the residual rounded tip to a more angular form by excision and closure of a small Joseph wedge excision.

In this case an additional T-shaped columellar strut was inserted to advance the colemullar base.

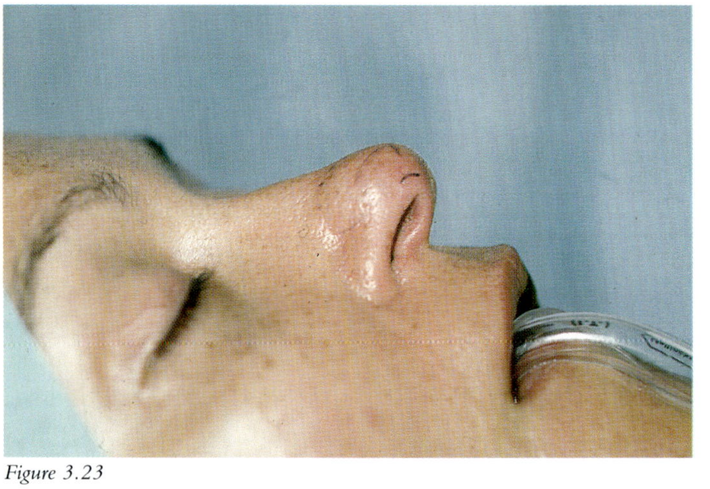

Figure 3.23

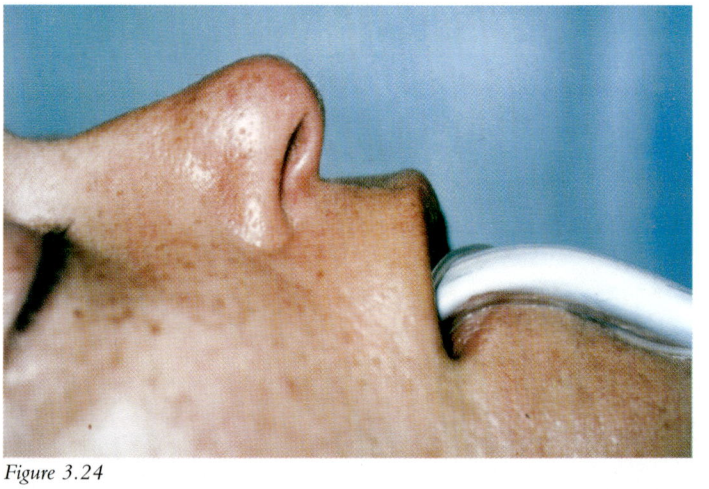

Figure 3.24

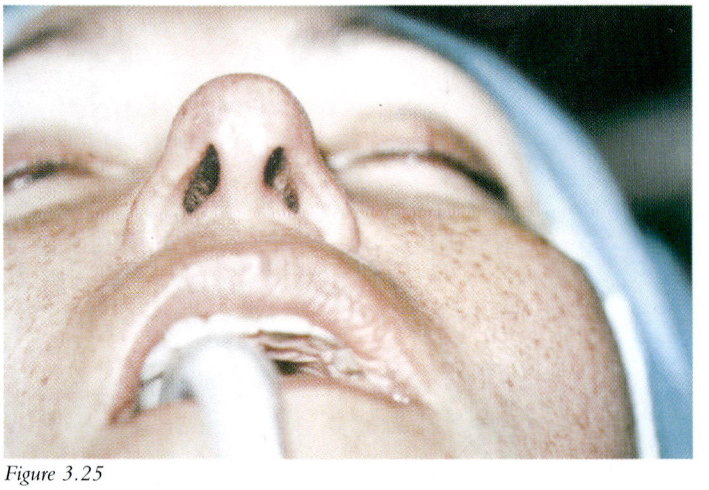

Figure 3.25

Bifid tip

This is really a variation of the broad tip. The divergent angle of the median crura is wide and the dome of the tip cartilages is rounded, forming a bilobular tip.

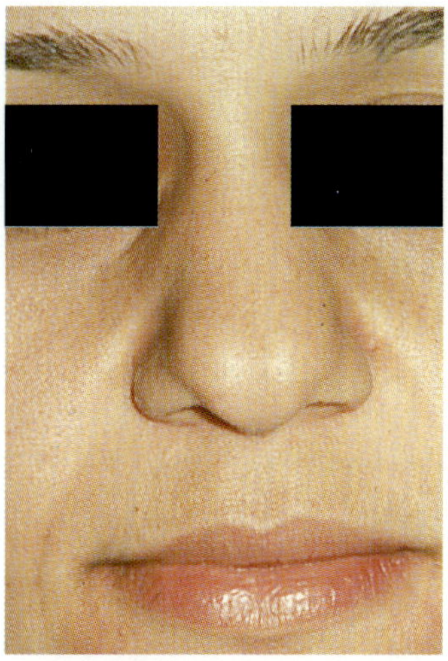

Figure 3.26a

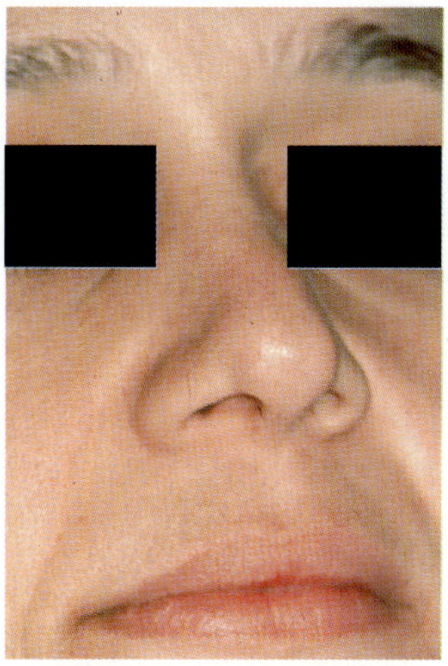

Figure 3.26b

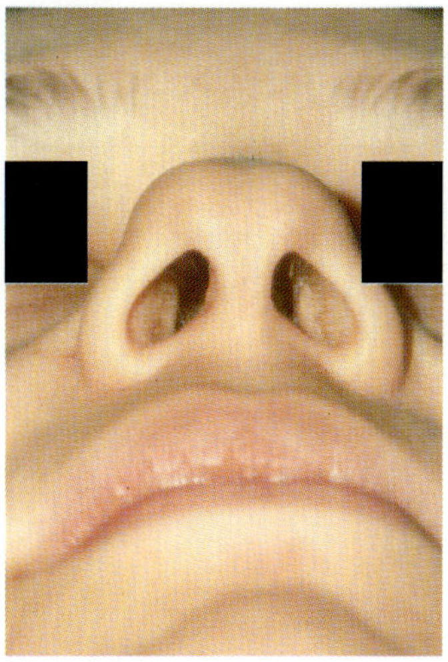

Figure 3.26

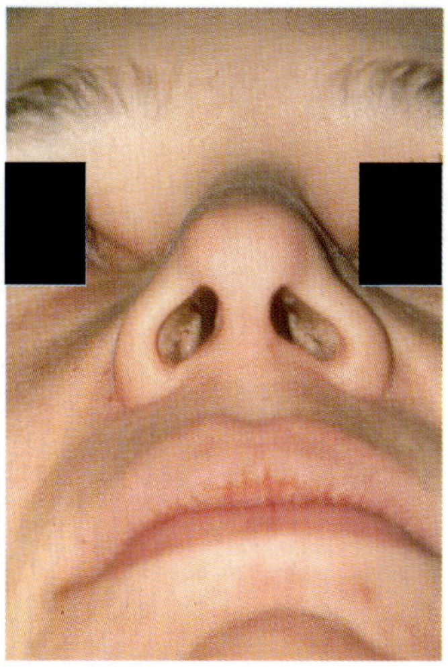

Figure 3.26d

Remove the excess cephalic portion of the lateral crus.

Expose the medial crura through bilateral rim incisions, and excise the intervening soft tissue.

Approximate the median crura with two interrupted 5.0 nylon sutures placed beneath the skin. A Joseph wedge excision may then be required to give angularity to the tip profile.

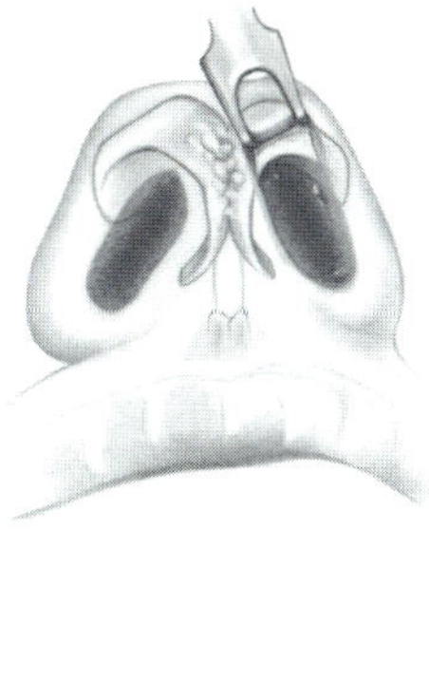

Figure 3.27a

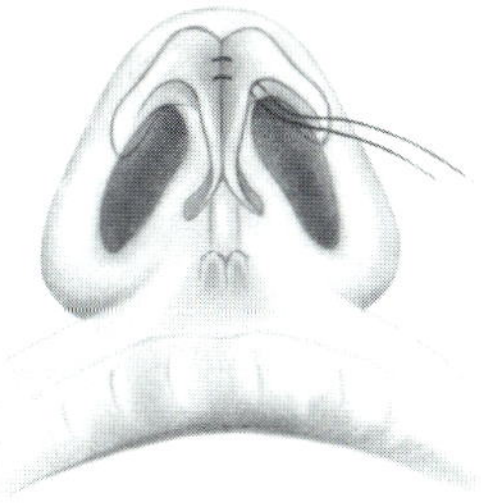

Figure 3.27b

Hanging tip

This term is used to describe a nasal tip that is either too long or lacks columellar support.

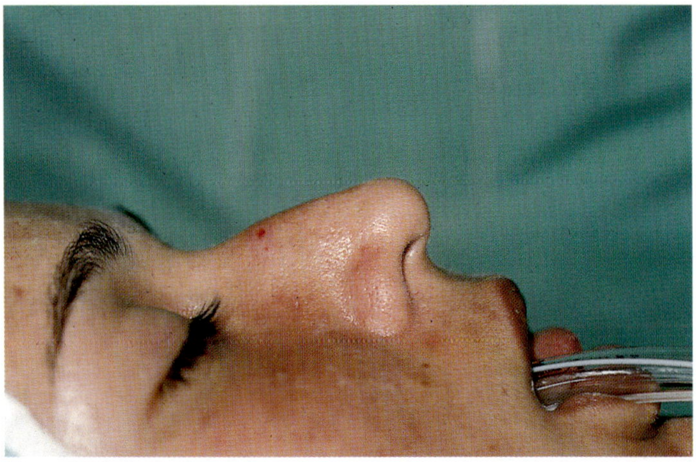

Figure 3.28

A short columella will pull down and lower the tip of the nose. In contrast a columella of adquate length which lacks skeletal support will cause the tip to rotate downwards; this is an essential component of a 'hanging tip'. Achieving the correct nasal length is a matter of aesthetic judgement, and is determined by basic rhinoplasty technique when the septum is shortened and angled (page 30).

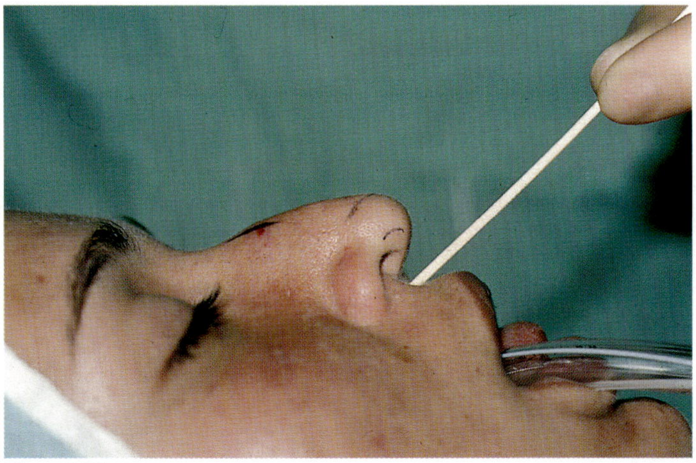

Figure 3.29

Columellar support is usually deficient if the anterior border of the septum or anterior nasal spine has been damaged — a common undiagnosed childhood injury.

A T-graft cut from septal cartilage adds skeletal support both to the columella and at its base.

Use the tip scissors to clear the soft tissues from the region of the anterior nasal spine. Use the opened scissor tips as a retractor while the cartilage graft is introduced down on to the maxilla.

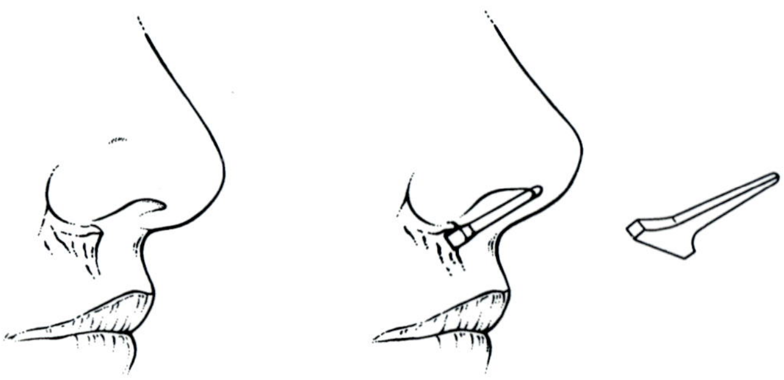

Figure 3.30

A second or even third layer of cartilage may be necessary.

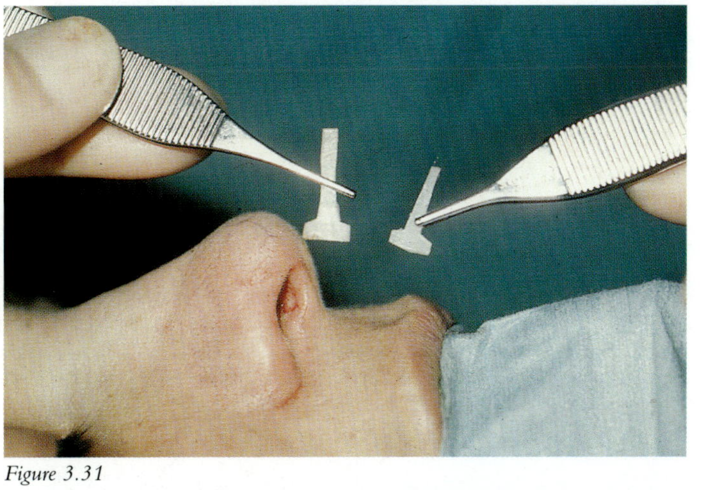

Figure 3.31

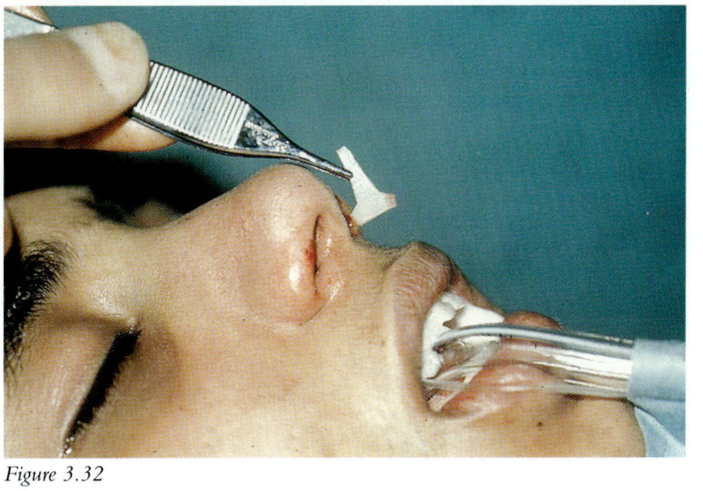

Figure 3.32

The vertical portion of the T cartilage is enclosed between the two skin surfaces of the membranous septum immediately posterior to the medial crura.

This is done by separating the skin edges along the posterior cut surface of the columella for about 3 mm.

Do not try to insert the cartilage between the medial crura because this is unnecessary and can cause unattractive widening of the columella.

The length of the arm of the T graft varies according to the amount of correction required, but usually extends up to the columellar lobular angle which is a feature that needs to be re-established.

Slight tunnelling of the soft tissues with the tip scissors at this point between the medial crura will provide a convenient pocket in which to insert the tip of the graft.

Close the skin with 4.0 catgut on each side and reassess.

It may be at this point that more graft is apparently needed at the columellar base. A shorter T graft can then be added and usually can be inserted using the same technique with the tip scissors, after one or more of the posterior catgut sutures have been removed.

In more extreme cases an onlay maxillary graft will also be needed and will be inserted before the T graft.

With tip scissors clear the soft tissues more widely from the anterior nasal spine, and out laterally towards the nostril bases and caudally towards the superior labial fornix.

There is usually sufficient septal cartilage to provide graft material. The thicker posterior septal cartilage is the ideal site.

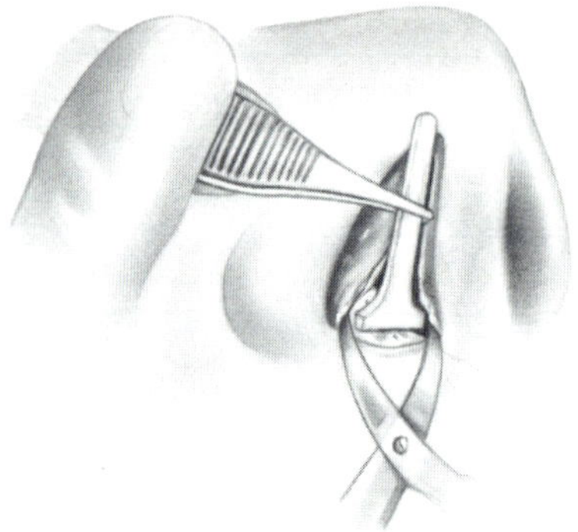

Figure 3.33

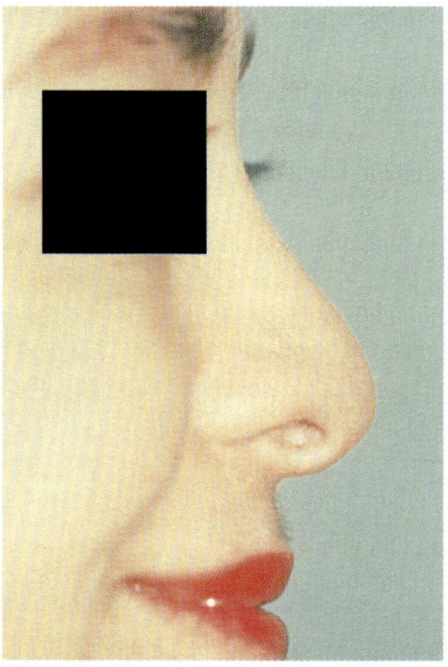

Figure 3.34a

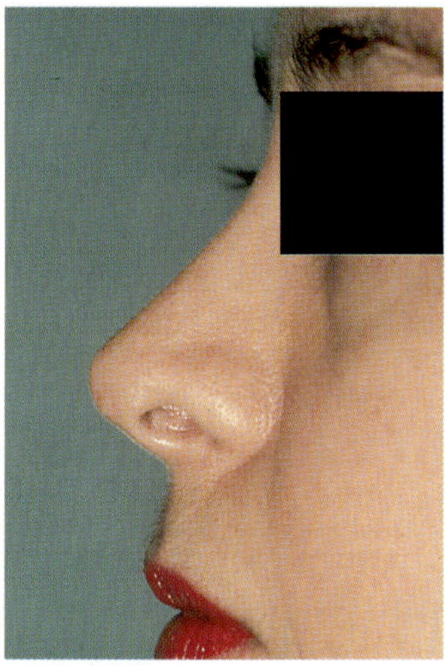

Figure 3.34b

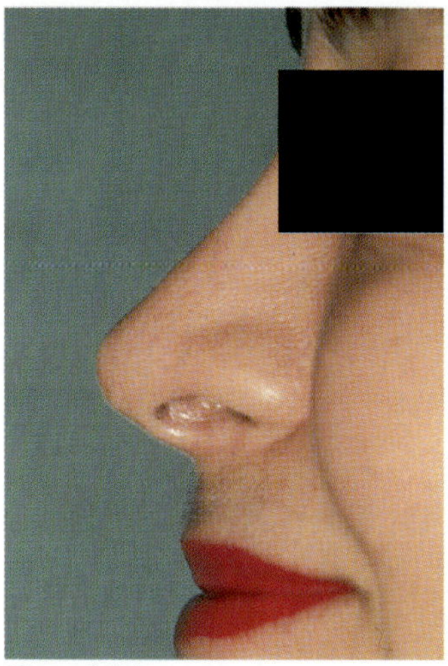

Figure 3.34c

Asymmetrical tip

Analyse the cause, which may be the direct result of asymmetry of the tip cartilages, or the indirect result of deflection of the anterior border of the septum. The technique for anterior septoplasty is described on page 71. If the asymmetry is the result of the shape and size of the tip cartilages it is preferable first to achieve as much improvement as possible using the basic rhinoplasty technique, and then to evaluate any residual deficiency. Most often a suitably designed tip onlay graft will compensate on the deficient side to raise, to define or to widen the underlying tip cartilage.

This evaluation and onlay graft are carried out only when the basic surgery and skin closure have already been completed.

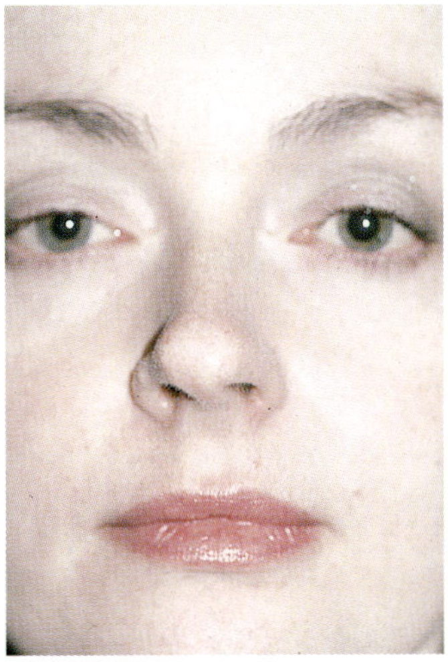

Figure 3.35a

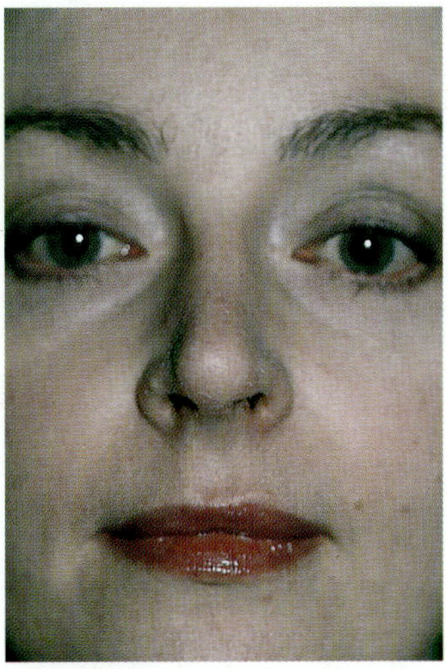

Figure 3.35b

Plunging tip

This may be associated with columellar retraction, a lack of columellar base support and a short upper lip.

Correction requires an understanding of the tip deformity as well as correction of associated defects which may also be present.

The primary deformity is caused by a long unsupported nasal tip which is pulled down on animation by powerful depressor nasi muscles (and to a lesser extent by the zygomaticus).

Associated deformities are treated as described under their individual titles.

Carefully examine the tip cartilage. The plunging tip cartilage may have a normal relationship to the skin in which case, remodel and refine the tip cartilage as described already (pages 32-34).

Fix the medial crura to the anterior edge of the septum with buried sutures of 4.0 catgut, having first dissected a space between the crura into which the septum can interdigitate.

In other cases much of the deformity results from the abnormal position of the lobular portion and lateral crus which lie close to the

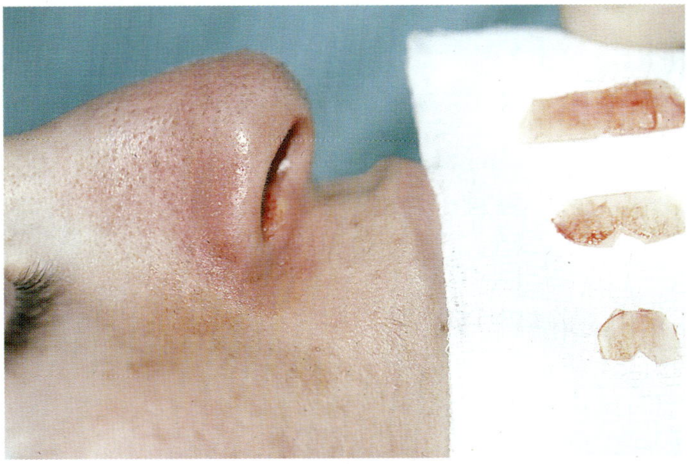

Figure 3.36

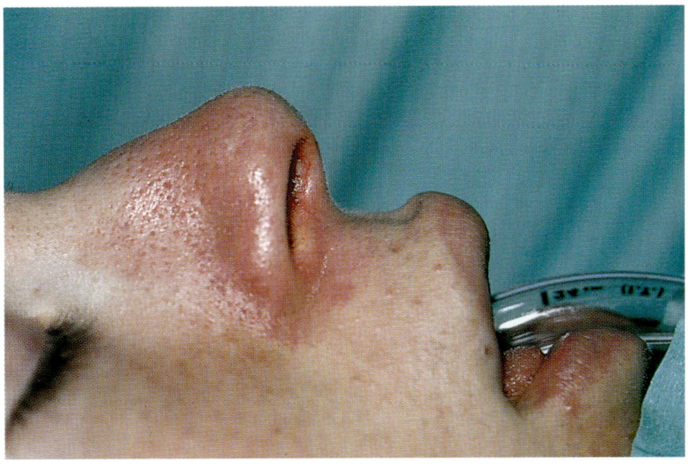

Figure 3.37

nostril rim, forming a steeply downward oblique slope to the cartilage.

Make a rim incision in the nostril margin. Through this expose the leading edge of the tip cartilage and incise a crescent-shaped strip. This creates a normal soft triangle of skin on the nostril rim, and also creates an improved shape to the lobular portion of the tip. In such cases elevation and transfixation of the medial crura to the anterior septum may not be necessary.

Septum and dorsum

Septoplasty or submucous resection frequently accompanies routine aesthetic rhinoplasty and may be indicated for correction of external deformity or internal deformity of the septum, or for the routine harvesting of a cartilage graft. Other cases associated with a respiratory malfunction and sinusitis may be performed in cooperation with an otolaryngologist colleague.

Routine submucous resection

This is best carried out after rhinoplasty dissection is completed and before suturing.

Anterior mucosal incision is carried out with a no. 15 scalpel preserving 1 cm of chordal and dorsal cartilage. If the deformity is localized, a larger amount of cartilage is retained. Make a vertical incision cautiously through the mucosa on the side of the septal deviation. Locate the correct plane of dissection under the perichondrium. This is less firmly attached inferiorly and dissection can be started more easily from this point.

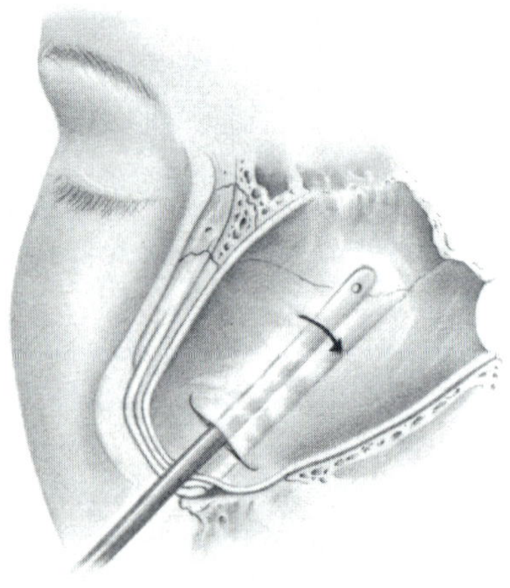

Figure 3.38

Push back the soft tissues along the edge of the mucosal incision until the correct plane is found. This is recognized when the shiny pale cartilage is exposed, and a clean plane of separation is entered. Dissection must always be carried out in this plane or the mucosal flap will be weak and torn too easily.

Use a Negus suction dissector to strip the perichondrium by gentle sweeping motions.

The incision is now extended cautiously through the caudal septum in a slightly oblique direction, but avoiding incision of the perichondrium or mucosa of the opposite side.

Reinsert the Negus dissector and gently strip the perichondrium of the opposite side.

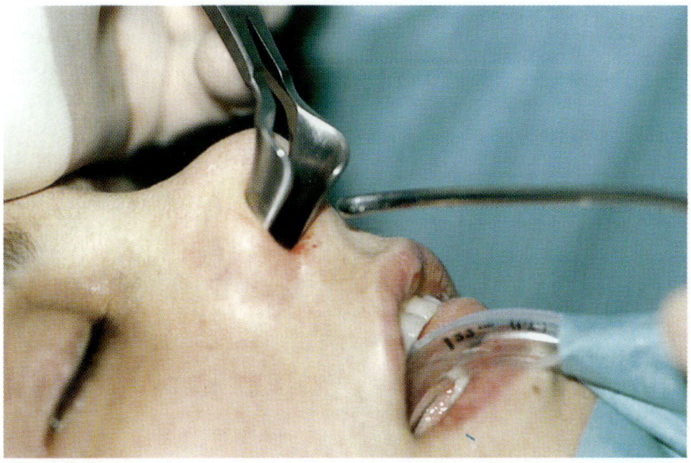

Figure 3.39

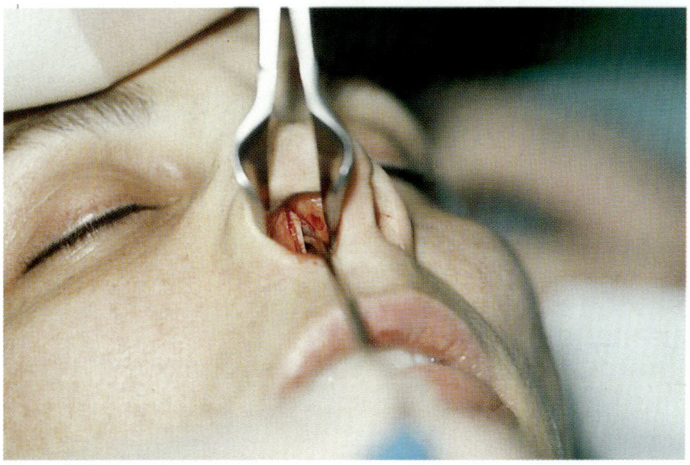

Figure 3.40

Before inserting a Ballenger knife start the cartilage incision with straight iris scissors to define the precise level and direction.

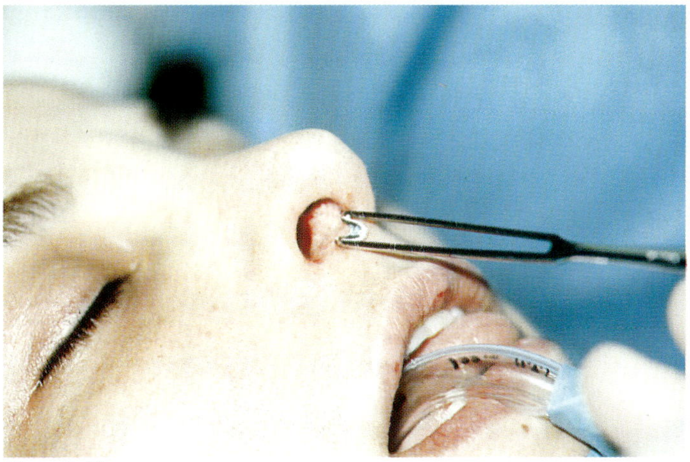

Figure 3.41

The Ballenger swivel knife is now inserted, extending the cut cephalad until the vomerine bone is reached, and then downwards and caudally to complete the excision.

When required a useful wider additional longitudinal strip of cartilage may be bluntly dissected out from the vomerine groove, providing material for a columellar strut if supplementary septal cartilage is needed.

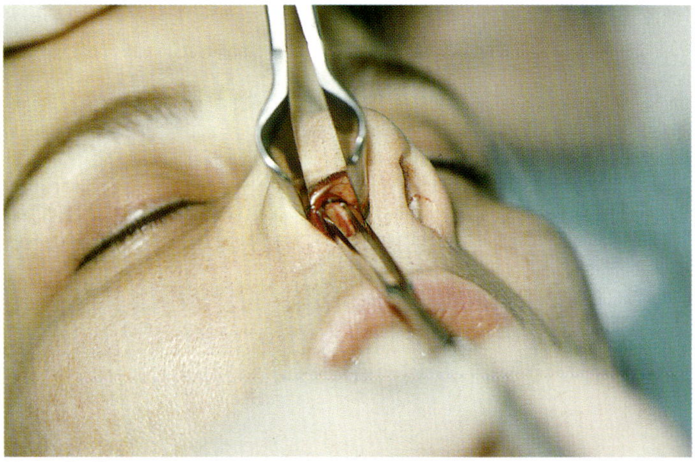

Figure 3.42

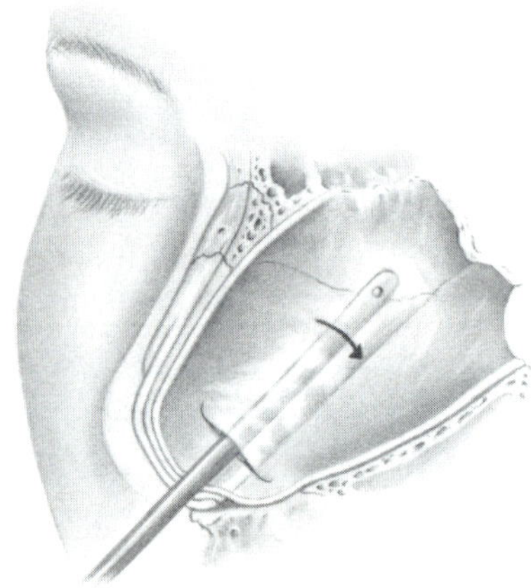

Figure 3.43

When indicated bony deformity or spurs involving vomer and the perpendicular plate of the ethmoid are then excised using a combination of dissection with a narrow (4 mm) osteotome and duck-billed Killian forceps. This technique is for the harvesting of cartilage grafts or the clearance of airway obstruction caused by septal deformity.

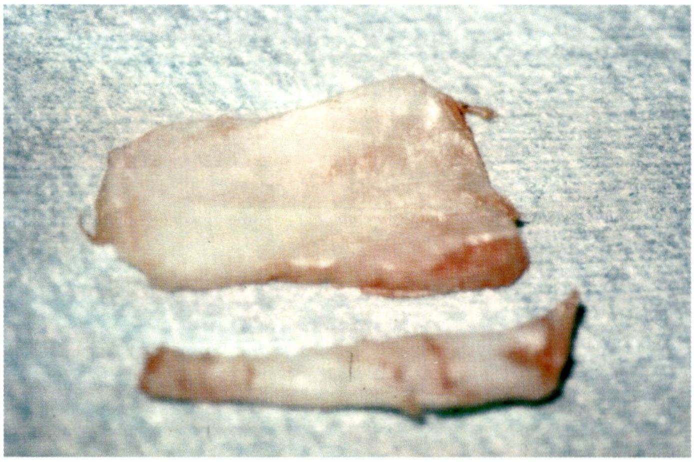

Figure 3.44

Anterior septal deviation

This involves the caudal portion of septum essential to support of the supratip region.

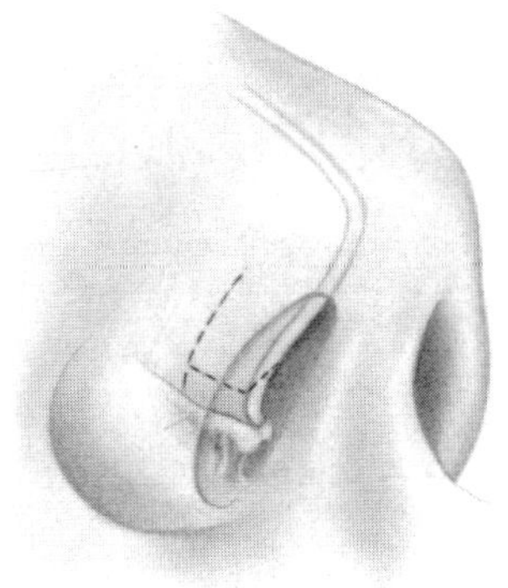

Figure 3.45

An extreme anterior deformity may be corrected when routine septal shortening is a necessary part of the aesthetic rhinoplasty.

In other cases, where the deviation is mainly adjacent to the anterior nasal spine, a bevelling excision of the prominent cartilage and even bone can be carried out without any need to cause septal shortening.

Where the whole anterior 1 cm of caudal septum is deflected, make an oblique incision with a no. 15 blade through the posterior septum, immediately anterior to the nasal spine, slanting the cut towards the side of the deflection.

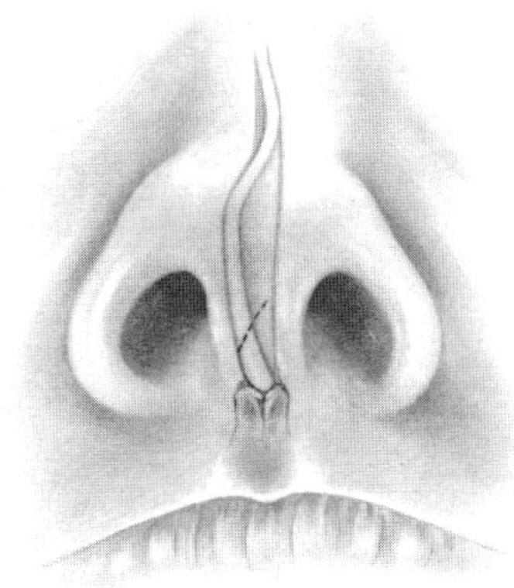

Figure 3.46

With the blade still in place now extend the cut through a right angle towards the dorsum for 0.5 cm which will weaken the spring resistance felt in the anterior deviated portion.

Gently grasp the caudal free edge of the septum lifting it upwards (anteriorly) so that the septum now 'flips over' the spinal portion and locks in a slightly over-corrected position. This is a quick, reliable technique which avoids need for awkward suturing through bone.

If there is residual fullness in the region of the anterior nasal spine, trim this cautiously with a rongeur.

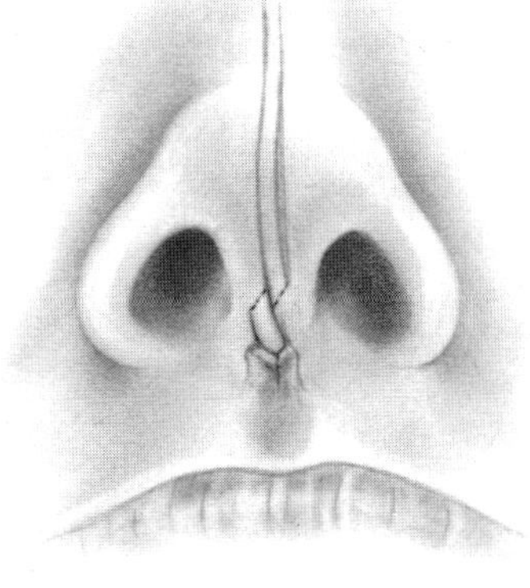

Figure 3.47

At completion of the rhinoplasty, closure of the mucosa using a circumferential suture will stabilize the caudal septum further and approximate the overlying soft tissues.

Occasionally it is necessary to stabilize the caudal edge of the septum further in its corrected position. This is done with a transfixation suture of 4.0 plain catgut brought out and tied over the skin of the nostril floor.

Spiral deformity of the caudal septum will be corrected only by subperichondrial stripping on the concave side and scoring of the cartilage. Initial incisions in the cartilage are made parallel to the contour of the deviation, and supplemented by diagonal cuts if further adjustment is needed.

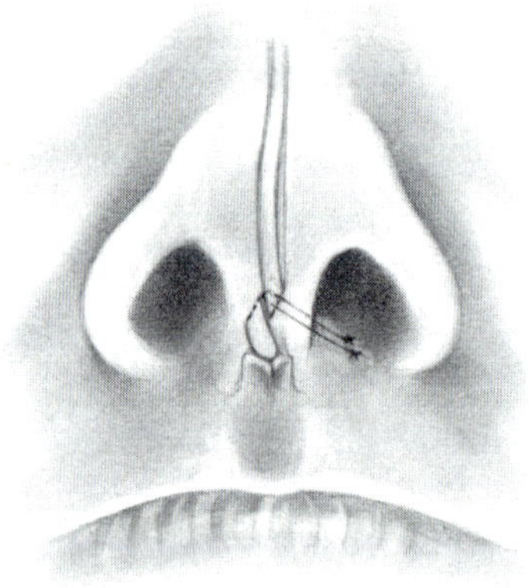

Figure 3.48

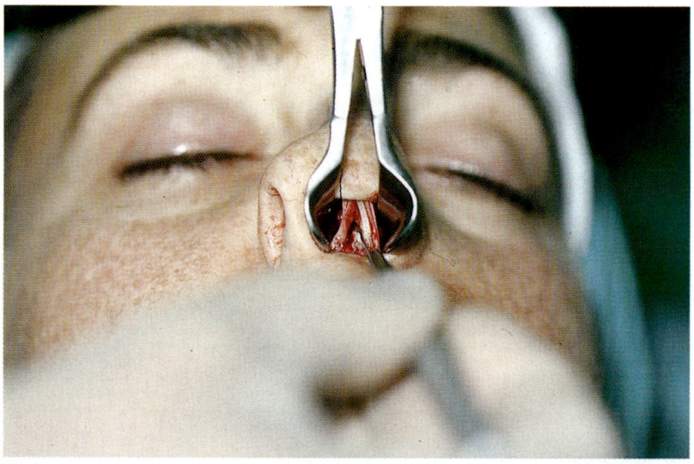

Figure 3.49a

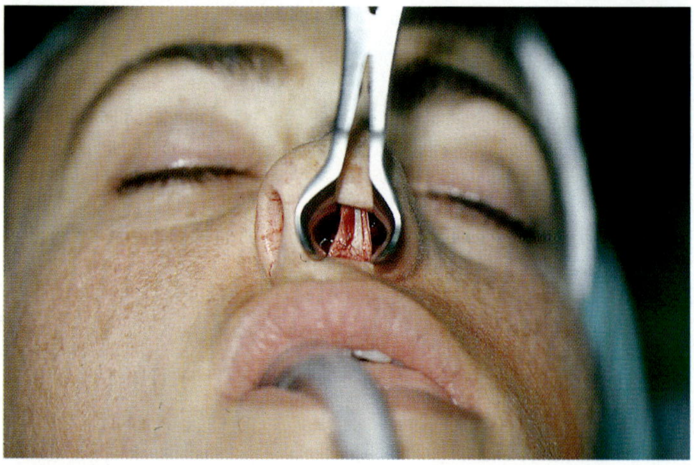

Figure 3.49b

Great caution must be taken to avoid excessively deep cuts penetrating more than half the depth of the cartilage, so that adequate stability of the cartilage is retained. In very severe or complex deformities subperichondrial stripping must be carried out on both sides to allow scoring of the septum in an additional concavity on the opposite side.

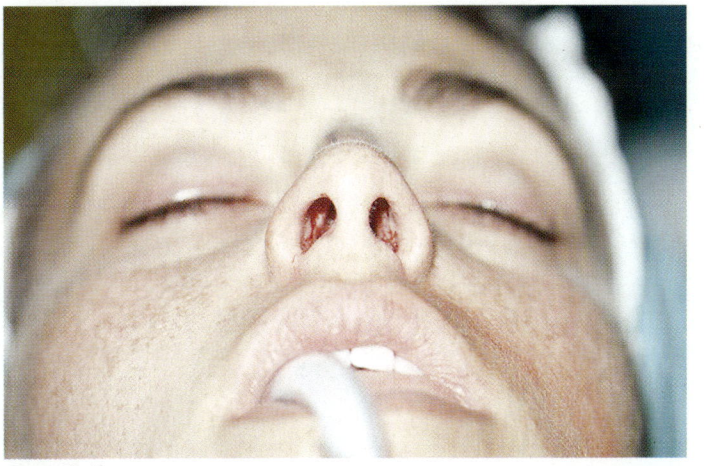

Figure 3.49c

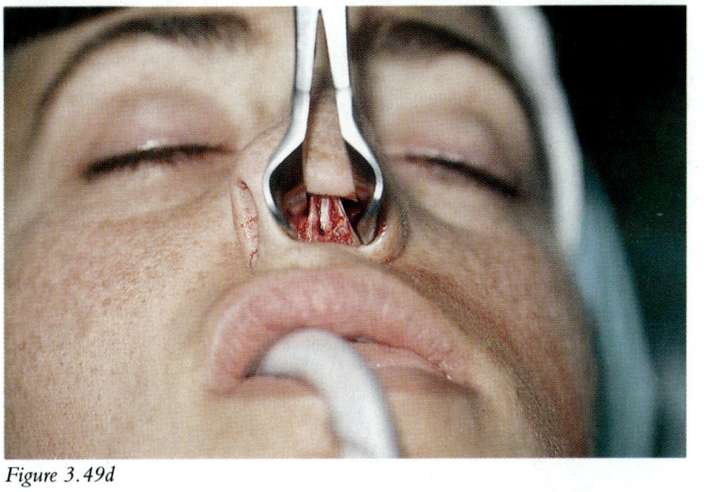

Figure 3.49d

A similar case in which another septum is secured with a catgut suture after correction of the deformity.

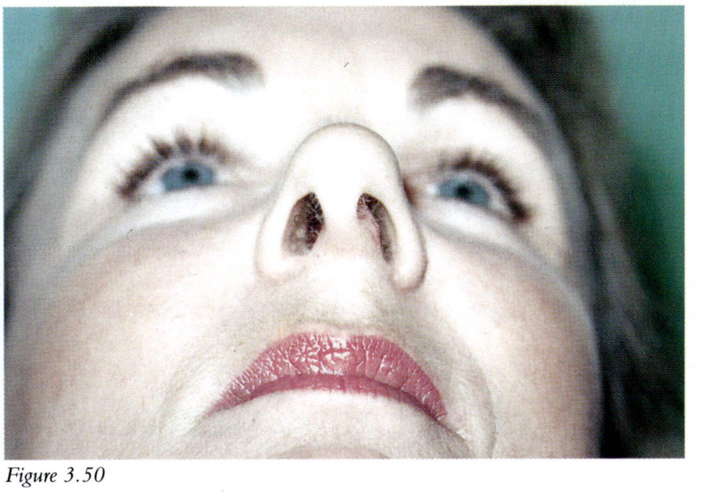

Figure 3.50

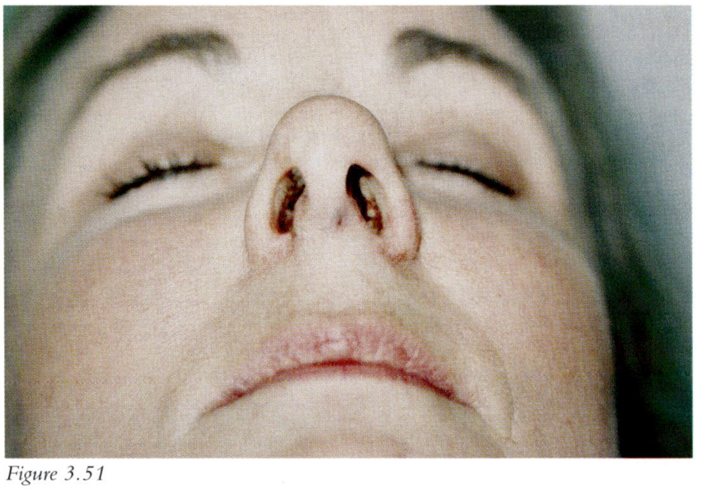

Figure 3.51

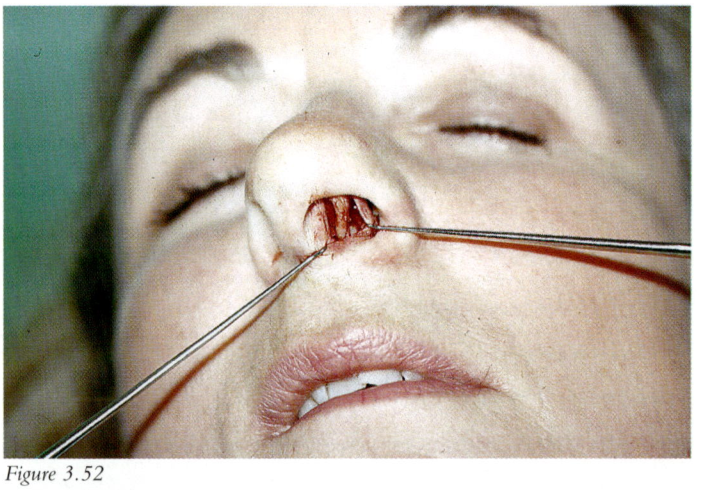

Figure 3.52

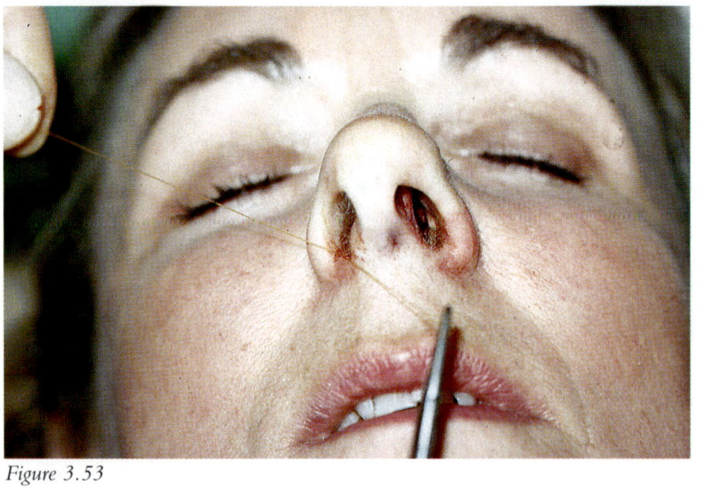

Figure 3.53

Dorsal deformities

Minor deformity can often be masked by inserting a thin cartilage graft subperichondrially on the concave side to fill out the depression. The graft usually remains stable in the dissected space.

If there is a tendency for the graft to drop down, a transfixation suture of 6.0 nylon can be inserted and tied externally without tension.

When the deformity is more marked as a result of septal deviation, subperichondrial stripping and cross-hatching of the concave side are carried out. This could be done for a simple C-shaped septal deviation. In more complex cases a spiral deviation or S-shaped deviation may require more extensive subperichondrial stripping to gain access to the whole deviation.

Following mucosal suturing the airways are packed with Sofratulle.

Whenever practical, I remove this from the wider airway after 2 hours, but retain it in (or repack) the side of the previously narrowed airway for 48 hours.

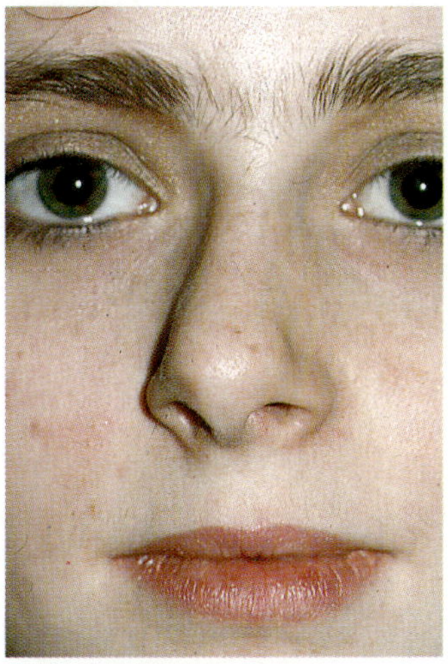

Figure 3.54a

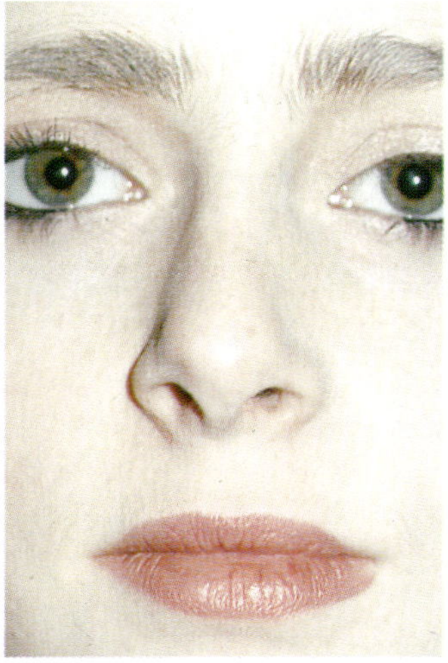

Figure 3.54b

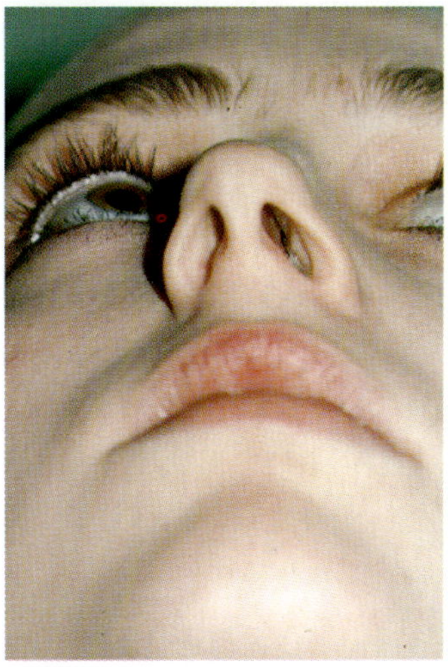

Figure 3.54c

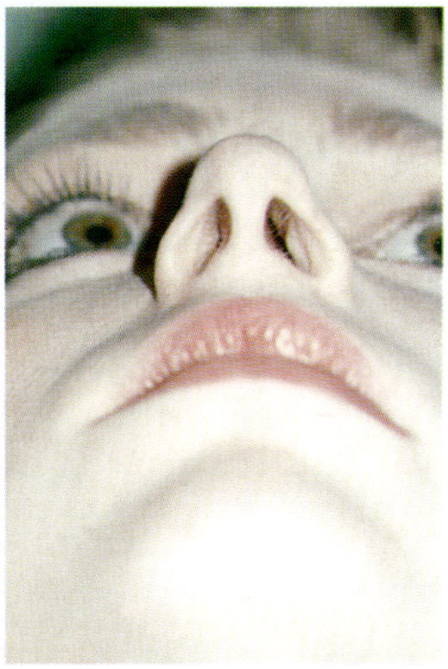

Figure 3.54d

Spiral (propeller) deformity

This creates a three-dimensional twisting deformity with both deviation of the dorsum and anterior septum. Complete skeletonization of the septal cartilage is required, and greater exposure can be gained by external rhinoplasty (if preferred), particularly if the nostrils are small.

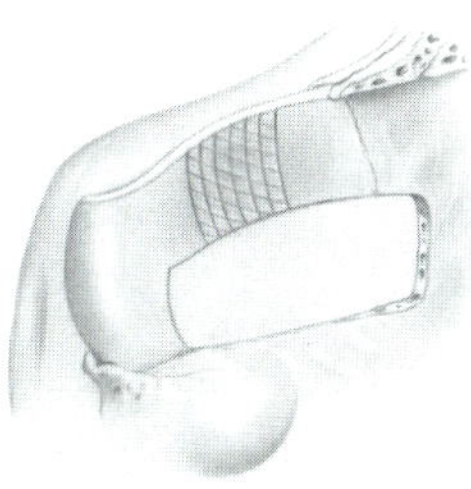

Figure 3.55

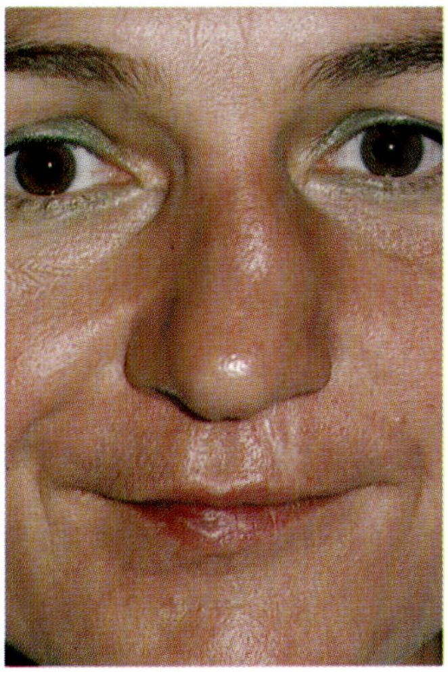

Figure 3.56

Expose the anterior edge of the septum through the membranous incision. In this area the perichondrium is very tightly adherent, so that extra care and patience are needed. Carry the subperichondrial dissection up over the dorsal edge until the septum is fully exposed.

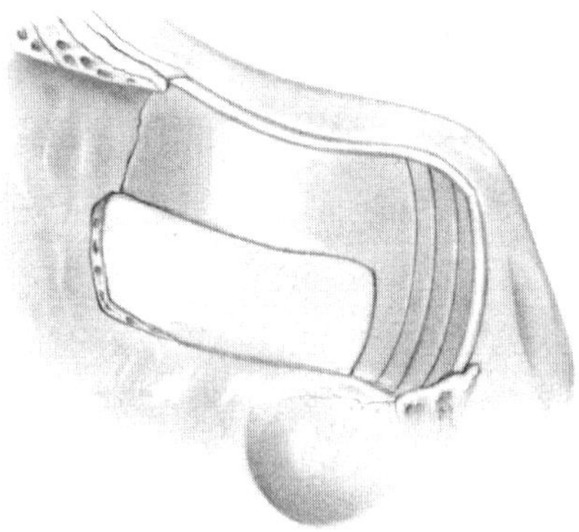

Figure 3.57

The concave surface is now incised superficially with parallel cuts along the contour of the deformity, usually at 2 – 3 mm distances. Further correction if needed, can be gained by incising diagonally to the initial incisions.

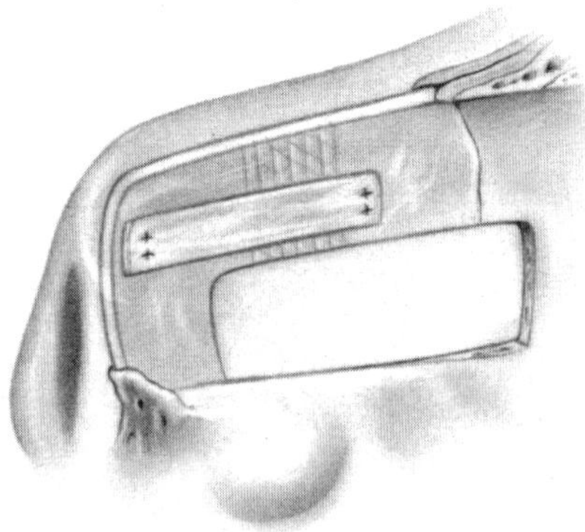

Figure 3.58

Turbinates

Hypertrophy causing mechanical obstruction is usually the result of thickening of the erectile mucosa which characterizes the inferior turbinates. This may often be noted on the widened (concave) side of a septal deviation. Cautery is a simple and frequently performed part of septoplasty or submucous resection, and is found to produce predictable correction. Turbinectomy is advocated by some surgeons with a high level of success and, contrary to previous belief, does not result in atrophic rhinitis.

Outfracture of a thin turbinate, using a no. 4 scalpel handle, is also a simple manoeuvre performed by digital pressure, although excessive force must not be applied.

When electrocautery is used in combination with correction of the deviation, the benefit is well maintained. In contrast, long-term benefit from electrocautery of the enlarged turbinate in allergic conditions, or when the septal deformity is not simultaneously corrected, will again lead to recurrent hypertrophy.

Columella

Both the columella and the alae are an integral part of the tip complex and when disproportion exists additional resection or adjustment may be necessary. This will have been part of the planned rhinoplasty but is performed after the more routine steps have been completed.

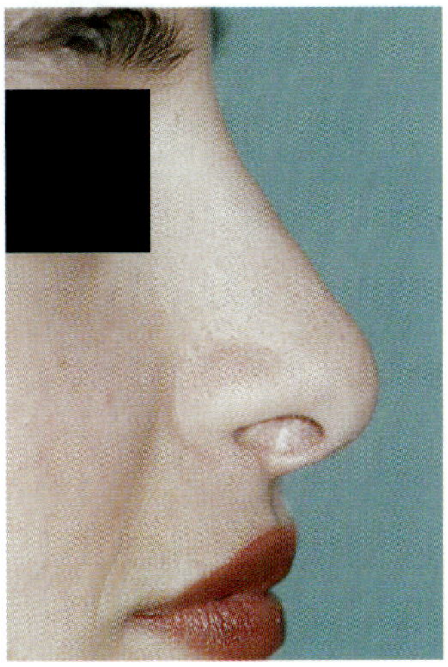

Figure 3.59

Columella disproportion

Hanging columella

This describes a columella that extends excessively far beyond the nostril margin; frequently it may be also associated with a drooping tip (see page 67). The columella normally lies 3—4 mm in front of the nostril margin.

If the deformity is mild, correct it by excising a suitable width of membranous septum and septal cartilage.

A more severe degree may result from the prominence of the medial crus.

Excise a narrow ellipse of skin and cartilage just inside the leading surface of the columellar margin. Make the taper very precise and also extend the incision up into the lobular portion of the tip to ensure a smooth and attractive angle to the columellar profile.

Close this incision with a continuous 6.0 plain catgut.

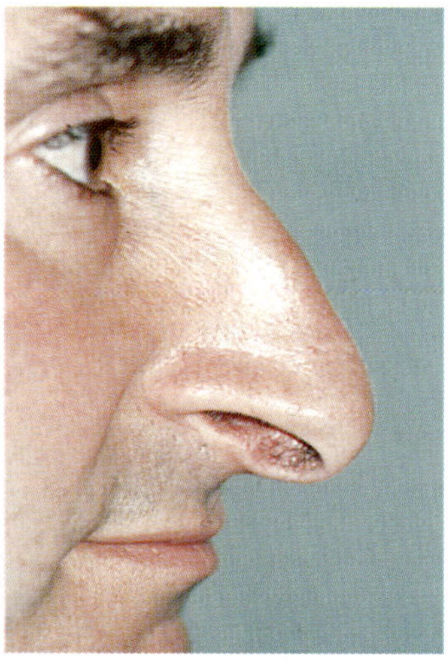

Figure 3.60a

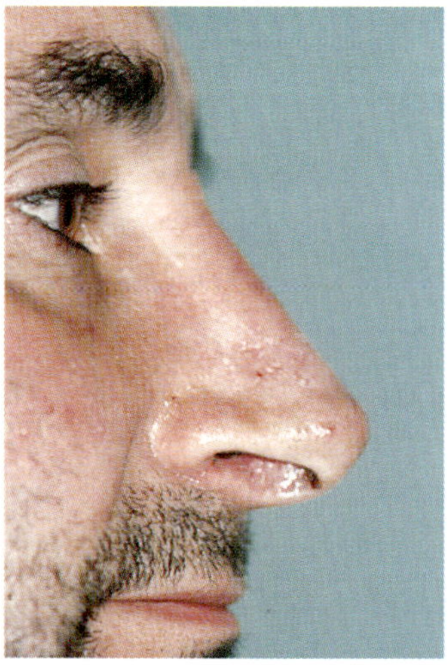

Figure 3.60b

Retracted columella

This can be caused by deviation of the anterior septum, which will then require correction.

More commonly the deformity will need correction by a septal cartilage graft.

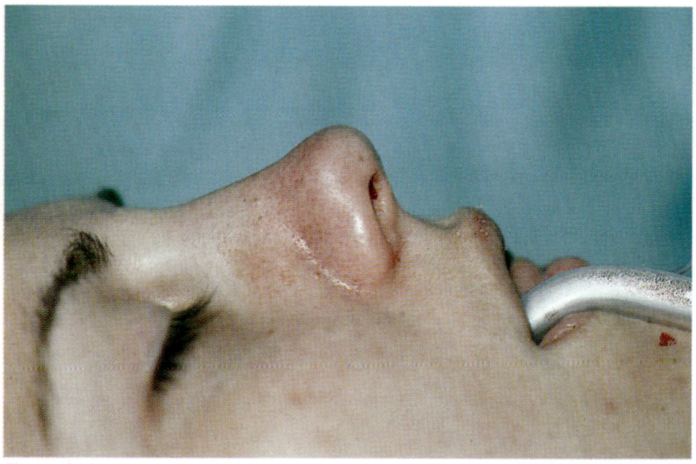

Figure 3.61

Free the soft tissues from around the anterior nasal spine and separate the medial crura just enough to allow skin closure later around the cartilage graft.
Carve a septal T-shaped graft of appropriate length (usually long enough to reach and define the columellar lobular angle).

Depending on the defect, one or more grafts will be required. Insert and suture these as described on page 64-66.

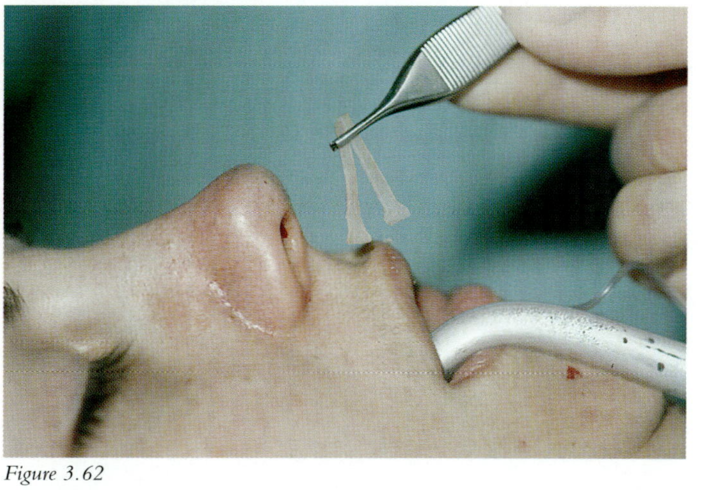

Figure 3.62

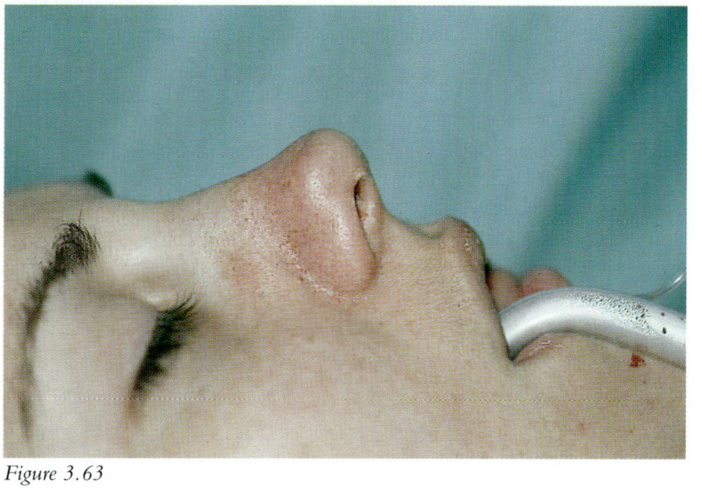

Figure 3.63

Long columella
Slight disproportion between an excessively long columella and short upper lip is corrected by stripping the soft tissues around the anterior nasal spine. This allows the base of the columella to slide downwards and to contribute to the upper lip length.
To gain additional shortening, excise the feet of the medial crus. The tightly adherent skin is carefully dissected off with fine dissecting scissors, and 3 – 4 mm of the cartilage excised on each side.
A similar segmental excision of the upper medial crus can be carried out (modified Lipsett technique), but is more applicable to tip modification problems.
If this results in a small fold of redundant skin, excise a wedge of skin at the level of the transfixation incision and in the direction of the nasal floor, which then avoids creation of an unattractive sharpened columella – labial angle.

Short columella

External skin incisions and scars are undesirable and instead every effort must be made to lengthen the columella by cartilaginous grafts.

Apparent shortness may result from either lack of tip projection or lack of skeletal support (maxilla) at the base of the columella. Surgical correction of these cases is described on pages 31-35.

True columellar shortness requires lengthening and stretching by an internal cartilaginous strut. Severe cases are best corrected by an umbrella graft, as described by George Peck. Tubulate a conchal cartilage graft (see pages 116-117) and insert this just behind the medial crura at their base. Separate the crura just enough to allow approximation of the nasal skin.

Tunnel through the anterior one-third of the space between the medial crura.

Elongate the columella by retraction with the thimble retractor and insert the graft. Tissue expansion by traction on the tip (with tip scissors not skin hooks) produces very valuable lengthening and enables a longer graft to be inserted.

The tip graft is then carved and inserted.

Less severe cases are often seen associated with a degree of lack of skeletal support at the columellar base; both defects can be corrected by inserting a T graft of septal cartilage.

Wide columella

When the depressor nasi muscles are large the columellar-lip complex is distorted, and the lip may appear to be pulled up into the nose: the columellar — labial angle is wide open and the columellar base wide. Use the skin hook to retract the skin edge and medial crus, and dissect out the bulky muscle. Once identified, clasp the muscle in an artery forceps, retracting and dissecting out the deeper portion of the muscle.

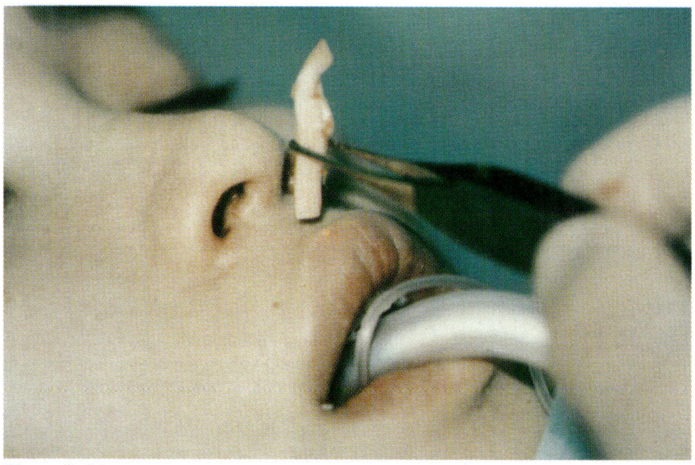

Figure 3.64

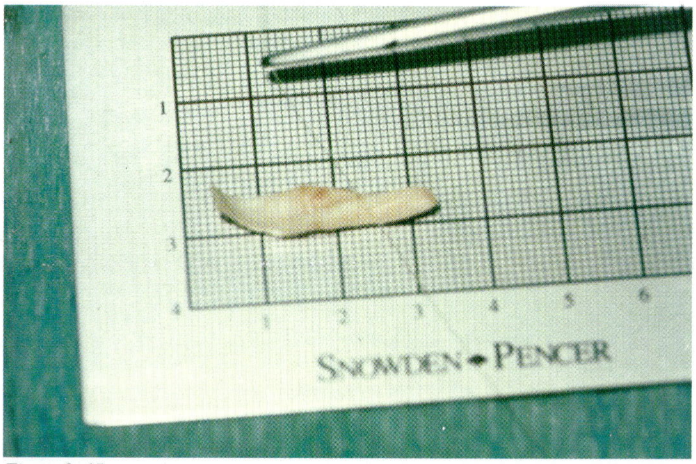

Figure 3.65

Repeat this on the opposite side. At the time of skin closure, use a catgut suture to approximate the medial crura and obliterate the dead space. The posterior end of this suture passes through the anterior border of the septum.

Alae

The most common deformity is flared nostril which will require excision of excess tissue at the alar base. A progressive realization of the wisdom of more conservative reduction rhinoplasty has also, fortunately, led to shorter incisions in the alar bases. Whenever possible avoid external skin incisions running out into the alar crease. This sebaceous wide-pored skin heals poorly with often conspicuous scars.

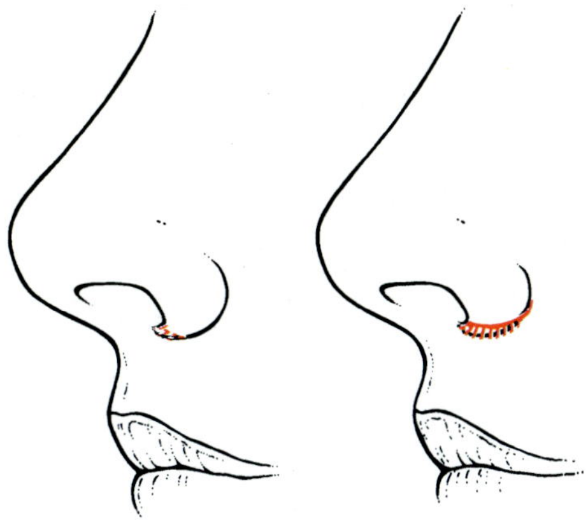

Figure 3.66

Always aim to place most if not all the incision on the inner or cephalic border of the nostril.

Other nostril deformities are thick nostril margins, retracted nostrils or wide bulky nostrils.

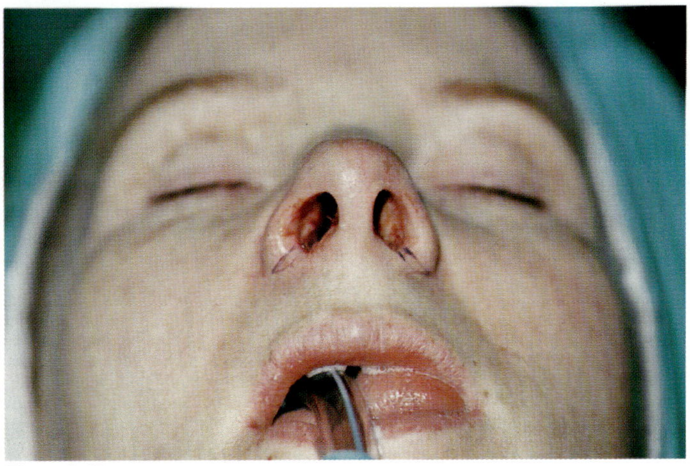

Figure 3.67

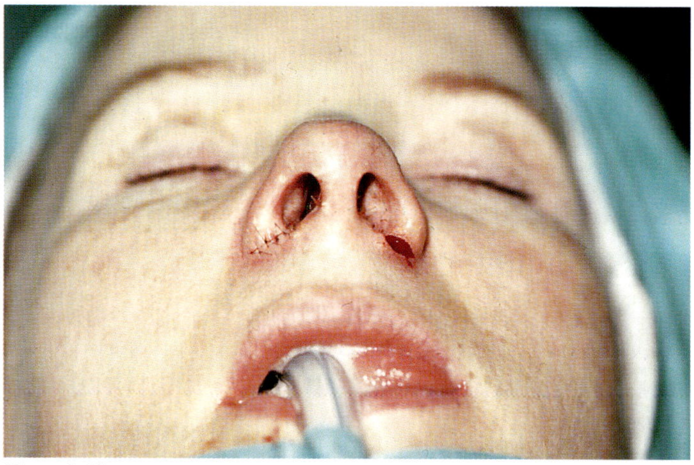

Figure 3.68

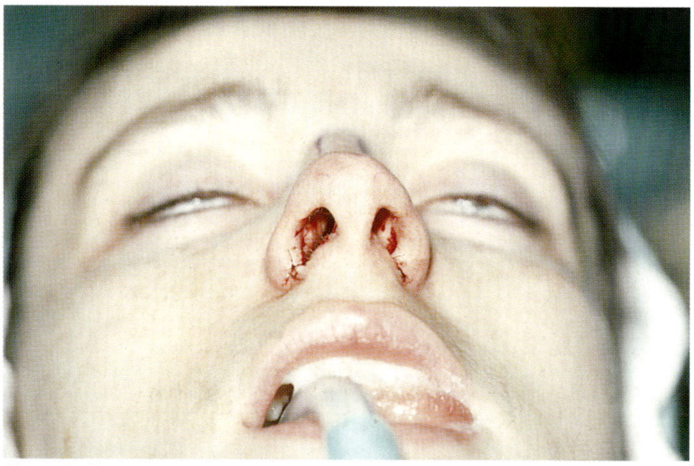

Figure 3.69

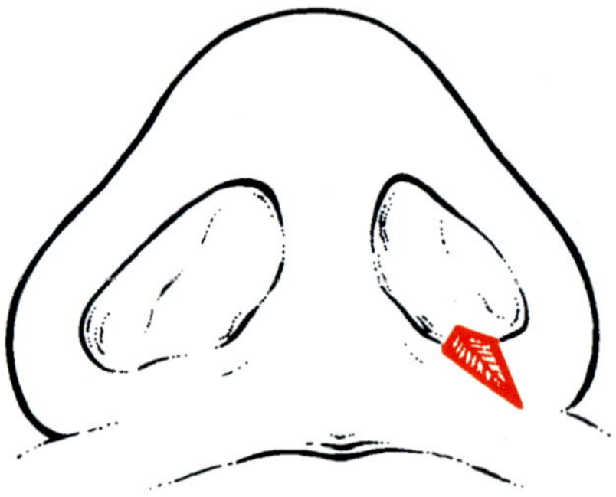

Figure 3.70

Flared nostril

Assess need for excision after the completion of rhinoplasty and suturing of the incisions. Skin closure will emphasize any excess flare or eversion of the nostrils.

Mark the proposed skin incisions so that skin closure will intersect the nostril sill obliquely. This prevents the stigma of notching of the healed scar.

Place the first suture at the nostril sill on each side to ensure that symmetry is present.

Close on either side with additional 6.0 nylon sutures.

The precise design of the wedge excision must be worked out for each individual case and may require unequal amounts of skin excision on the two sides.

However, always plan to try and restrict the skin incision to within the inner and cephalic margins of the nostril, to avoid a visible scar stigma.

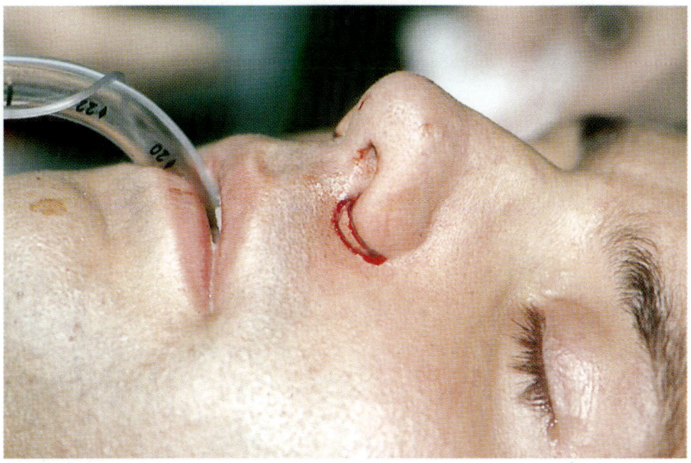

Figure 3.71

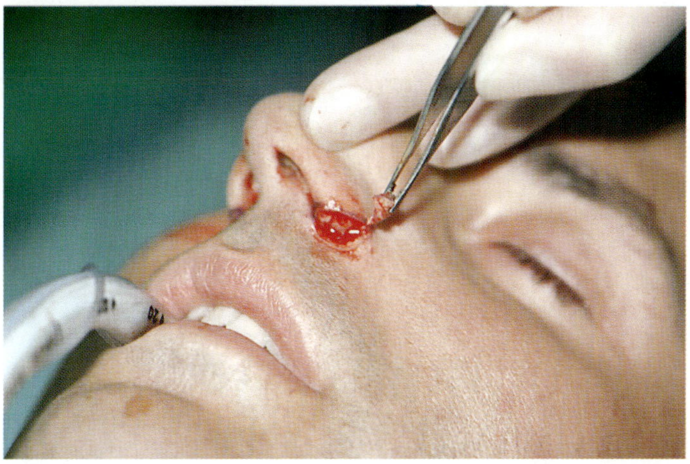

Figure 3.72

Thick or drooping nostrils

Wedge excision, as described by Ralph Millard, gives an elegant refinement and correction of this defect.

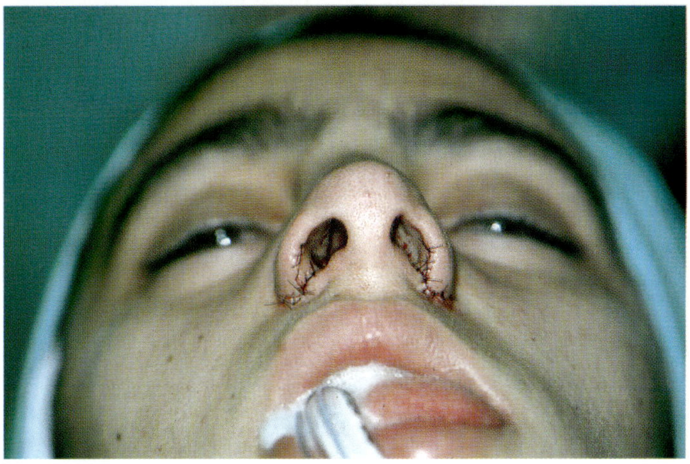

Figure 3.73

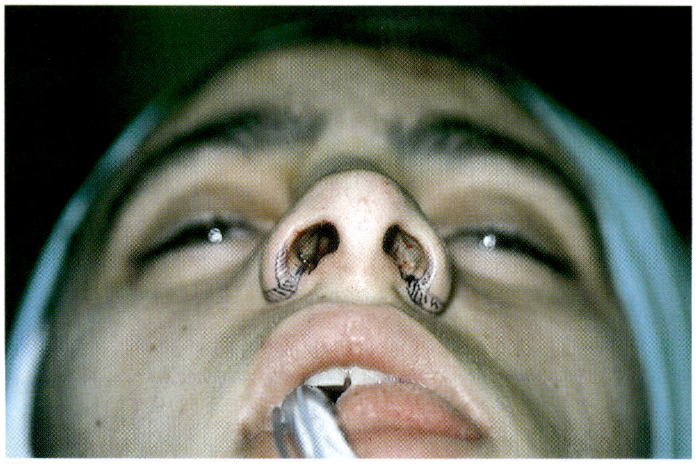

Figure 3.74

Mark the skin very accurately so that after skin closure the scar will lie concealed on the inner aspect of the nostril.

A combination of filleting of the nostril margin and alar base resection is often effective. Close the marginal incision with a 6.0 nylon running suture.

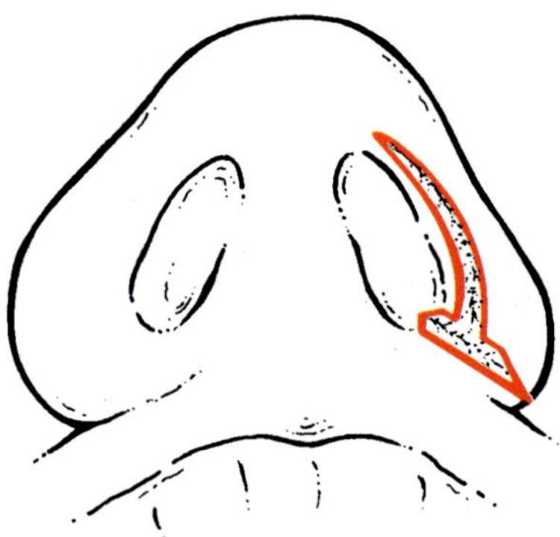

Figure 3.75

Retracted nostrils

This deformity can occur primarily, but more commonly it is a feature of secondary nasal deformity resulting from excessive excision of lateral crus and skin lining.

The technique of Rudi Meyer is favoured and gives a delicate and natural appearance to the advanced alar rim.

Incise the nostril lining skin about 4 – 5 mm inside and parallel to the outer margin.

Undermine and unravel the skin so that it can be advanced forward. Make this incision longer than the apparent defect so that a smooth outline is achieved.

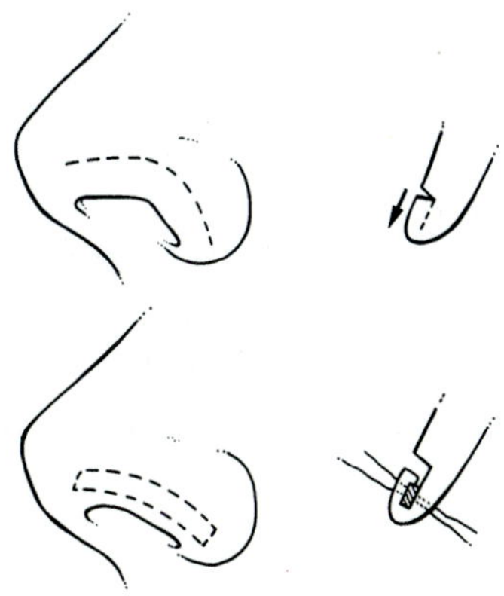

Figure 3.76

Insert a suitably sculpted septal graft into the bed of the wound. Slot this cartilage into pockets at either end so that it remains securely in place.

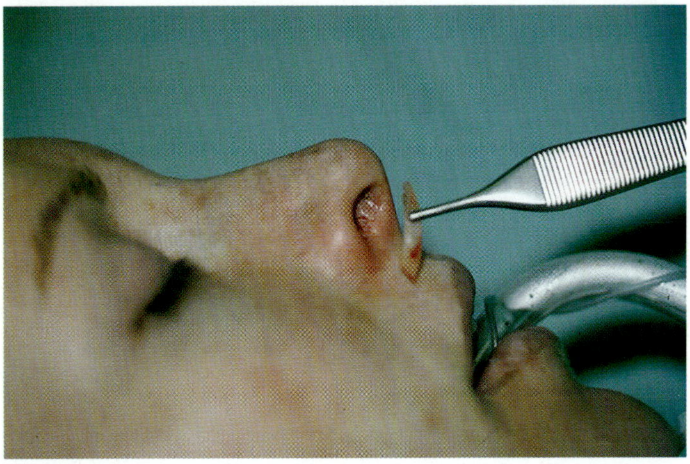

Figure 3.77

Maintain the skin and cartilage in place with gentle compression of the forceps, at the same time inserting two mattress sutures through skin and cartilage graft, tie these lightly. The graft should lie well forward in the cavity, covered by the unfurled skin lining.

A narrow raw surface remains and there will be rapid secondary healing.

Sutures are removed after 8 – 9 days and antibiotic ointment applied to the nostril incisions twice daily.

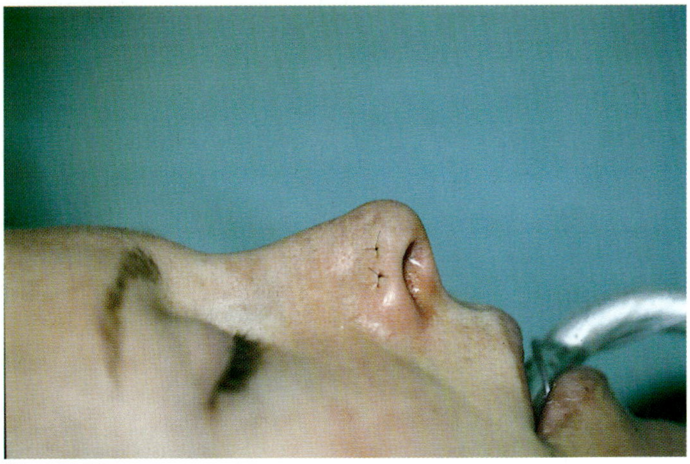

Figure 3.78

Part IV

SECONDARY RHINOPLASTY

Secondary Rhinoplasty

Introduction

Secondary rhinoplasty can be one of the most challenging problems in aesthetic surgery; in addition, the patient's resentment and possible process of litigation make a careful assessment and approach to treatment essential. Do not embark on treatment if litigation is pending, and be sure that you clearly inform the patient of the limitations of what you can achieve.

The timing of surgery is important and an interval of at least 6 months must be allowed for resolution of scar and swelling. Reassessment at this time may indicate need for further delay, and the patient may find this hard to accept. Sympathetic reassurance, careful examination and planning will help the patient to understand the problem better and to accept your professional judgement.

Choice of graft material

Bone, cartilage or dermis each have a suitable application. Always use autogenous material which will be well tolerated in spite of the scarring and diminished vascularity. Never use alloplastic materials in such unfavourable conditions. Choice and application of autogenous materials are illustrated for each anatomical area.

Whenever available, it is better to use the septal cartilage than the conchal cartilage. It can be carved to a more precise degree, bevelled to a required curvature, and its tensile strength is better suited for grafts to the columella and nostril.

When the septum is not available (previous surgery or injury) the conchal cartilage will provide alternative material. The technique is described on page 97. Excellent regeneration of cartilage and a far superior aesthetic appearance to this donor site is obtained if the anterior perichondrium is preserved.

Planning treatment

Careful examination and planning will generally expose a complex mixture of both aesthetic and functional problems requiring treatment, many of which may not have been recognized by the patient. For this reason staged treatment is sometimes necessary, although the subsequent operation is usually smaller and can be done under local anaesthetic, as an outpatient, a few months later.

For clarity the anatomical areas of the nose will be considered separately, although in practice the surgeon can expect to encounter a variable combination.

Dorsum

Collapse, excess removal of bone and asymmetrical defects will each create a variable degree of saddle deformity.

Grafts to the dorsum of the nose

Dermis grafts

Minor irregularity of the dorsum This is best treated by smoothing with a rasp and then masking or augmenting with a dermis graft.

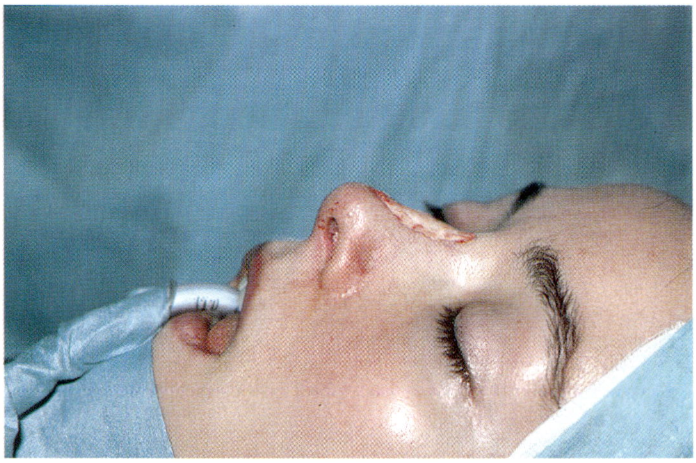

Figure 4.1

Trim the dermis with scissors to the required shape and size.

Insert the graft and suture in place with the smoother, more vascular, superficial dermis on the outside.

Insertion is quick and precise using the harpoon technique.

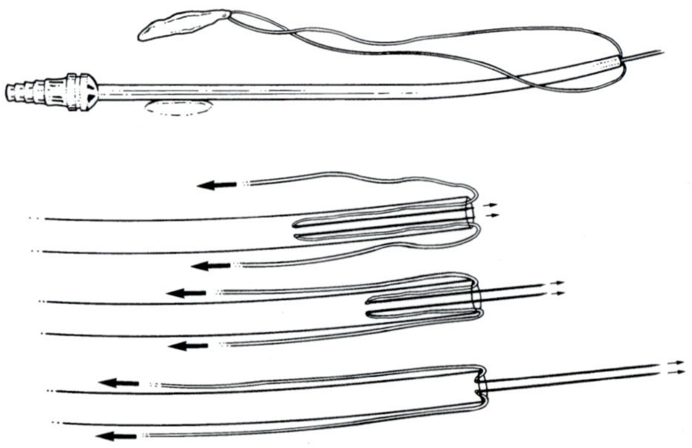

Figure 4.2

First pass a double-ended 4.0 suture with straight needles through the cephalic end of the graft.

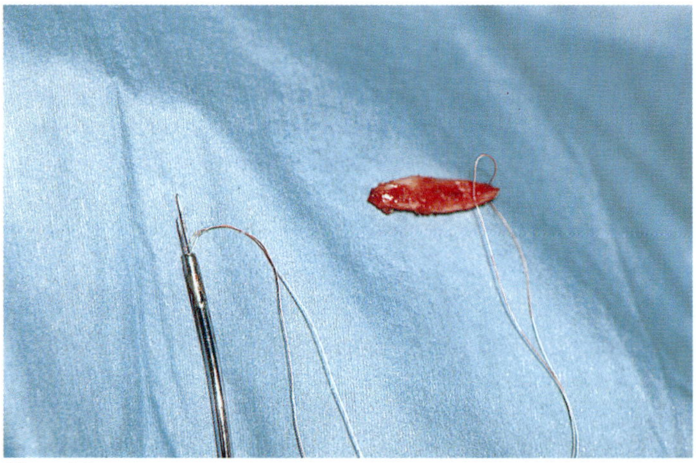

Figure 4.3

Load the needles into a narrow nasal sucker (switched off) with pointed ends presenting.

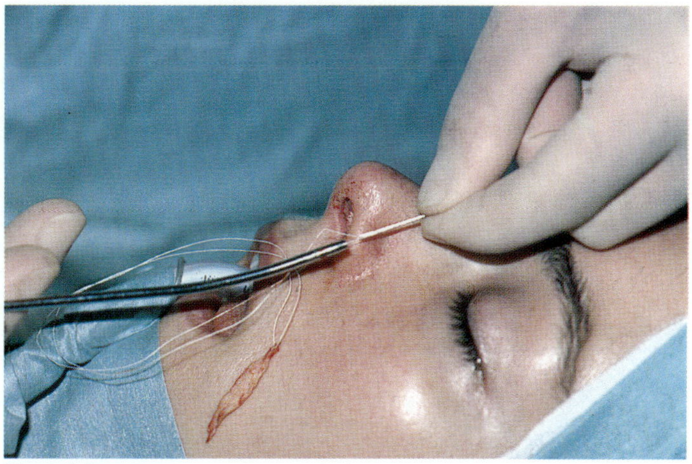

Figure 4.4

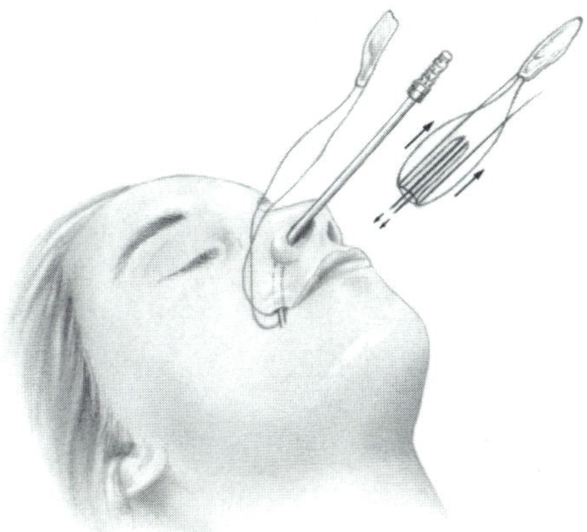

Figure 4.5

Pass the sucker up the nose to the desired exit site for the needles.

Apply gentle traction on the double sutures which will propel the needles through the skin.

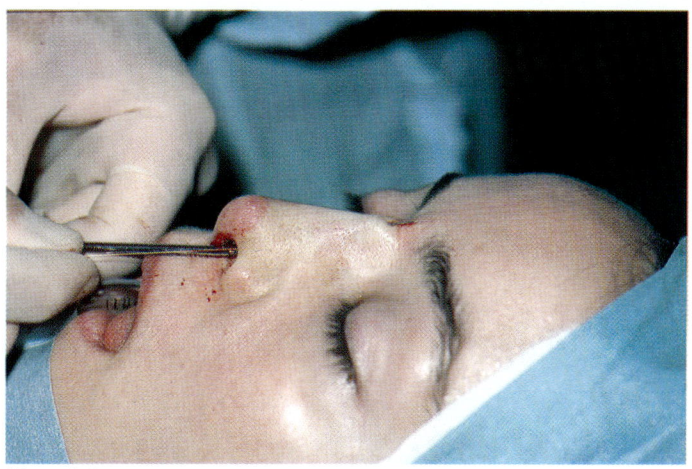

Figure 4.6

Draw the needles out through the skin, so drawing the dermis graft into place. A second suture at the caudal end is not usually necessary.

Tape the suture to the skin and trim off the excess.

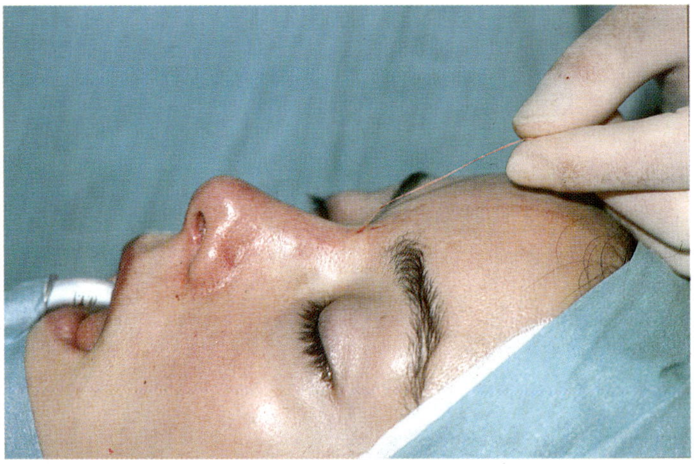

Figure 4.7

Before and 6 months postoperative.

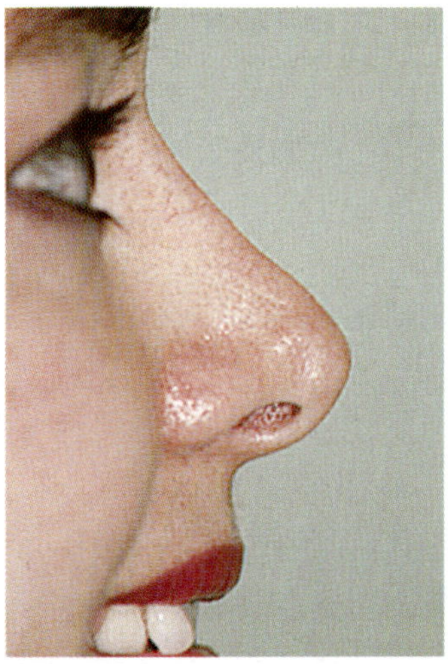

Figure 4.8a

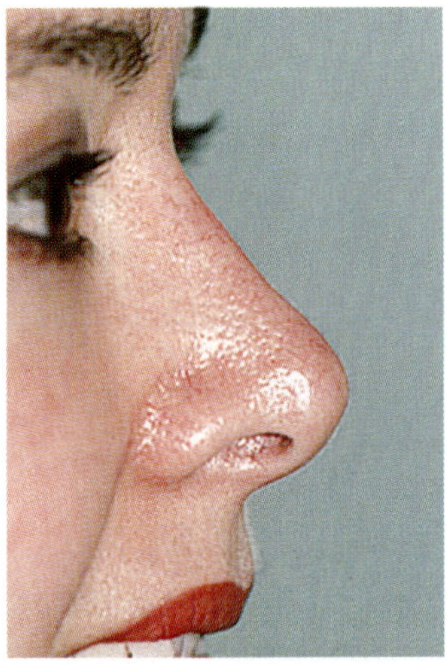

Figure 4.8b

Bone or cartilage grafts

In very large defects a bone graft from the iliac crest or calvarium may be preferable, but the rigid graft feels unnatural to the patient and is now less popular than in the past. Absorption of the bone graft can also occur.

In many cases a single layer of cartilage is sufficient, but when needed shorter less perfect pieces may be added on the deeper surface and secured with a fine plain catgut or collagen suture of 5.0 or 6.0.

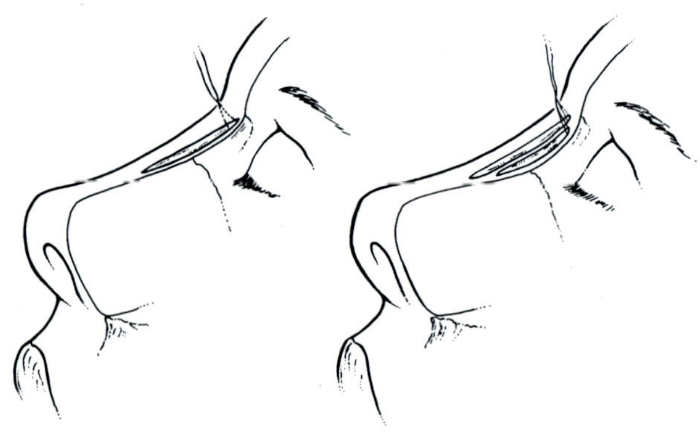

Figure 4.9

Minor saddle nose deformities

Depressions of up to 5 mm can be satisfactorily and conveniently filled by a cartilage graft carved to a precise shape and size.
Secure the graft to the overlying skin with a fine monofilament nylon at both ends, secured by Steristrips.

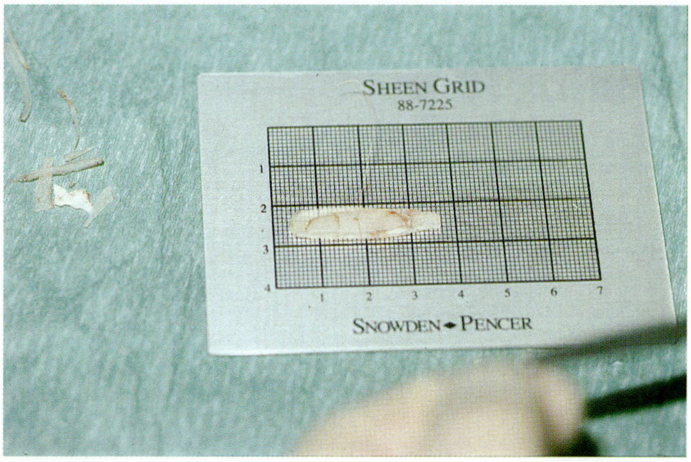

Figure 4.10

In this case three layers of septal cartilage were used to augment the dorsal profile.

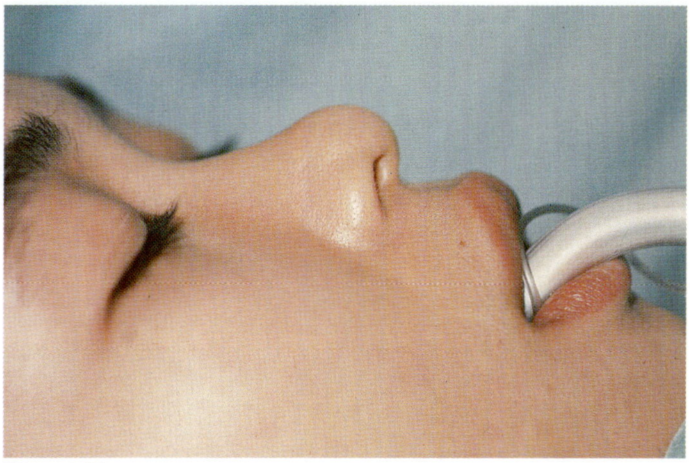

Figure 4.11

The tip has also been elevated by an umbrella graft (see pages 35 and 80).

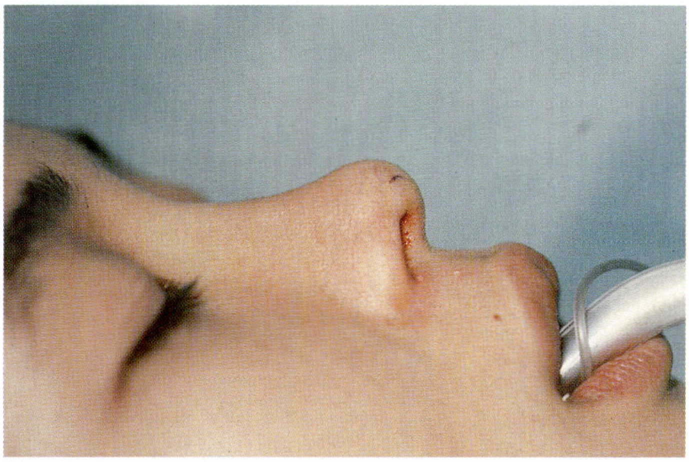

Figure 4.12

Severe saddle deformities

Airway obstruction is more commonly a problem in the middle vault, and treatment is described under this heading.

Whenever possible cartilage is preferred to bone because this will be less rigid and feel more natural to the patient. A combination of septal and conchal cartilage may be needed to gain sufficient bulk.

Long dorsal depressions involving mainly bony deficiency can also be corrected by a suitably sculpted iliac bone graft, as in this example. If accurately fitted it will be stable and not require pin fixation.

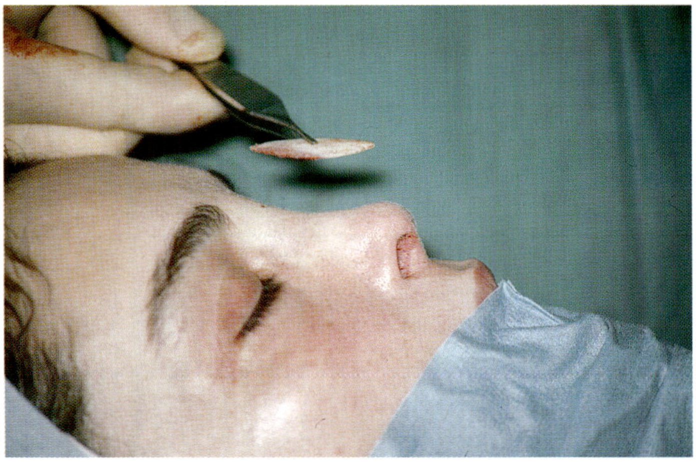

Figure 4.13

Rarely a costal cartilage graft is used when insufficient septal and conchal graft is available. (A previous iliac bone graft had absorbed.)

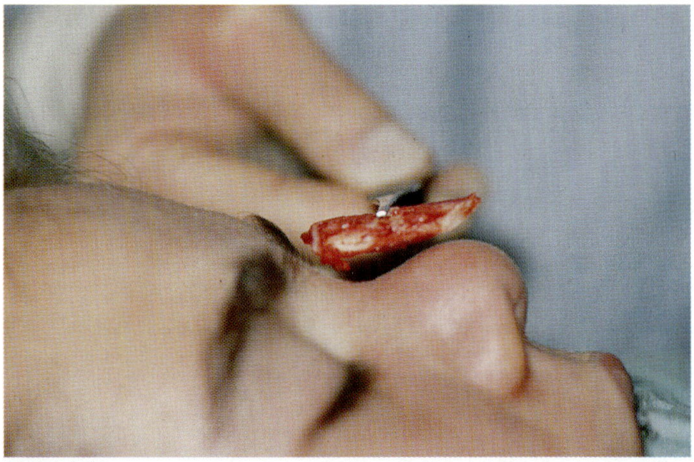

Figure 4.14

Before and immediately following insertion of the costal cartilage graft. This fits snugly into the dissected pocket and is stable without need for pin or suture fixation.

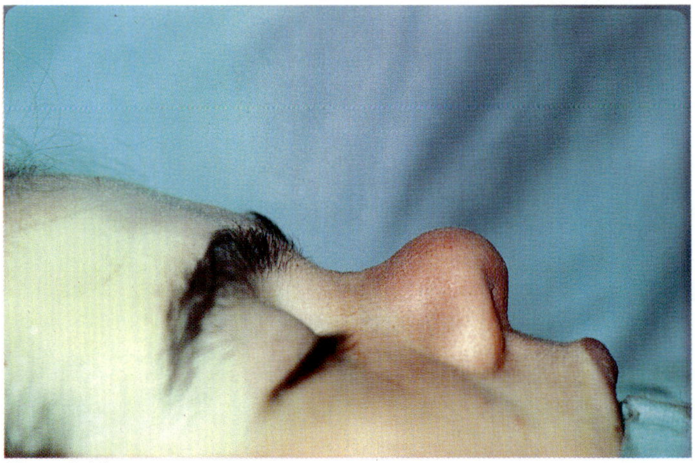

Figure 4.15a

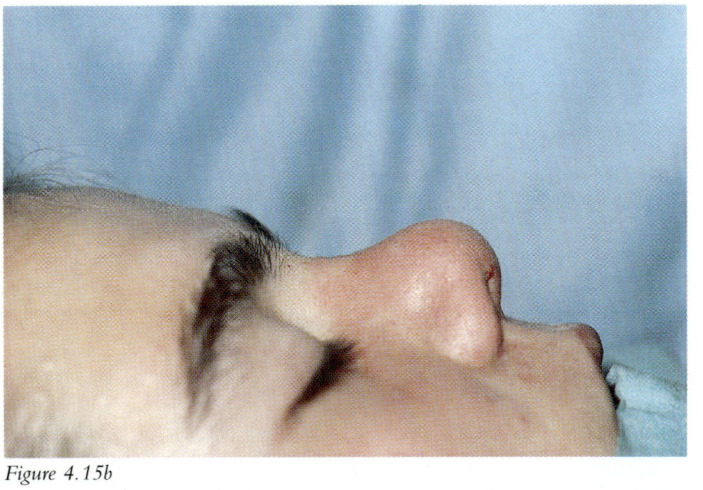

Figure 4.15b

Harversting the graft

Septum (see also page 68, Techniques of SMR)

Both for stripping the mucoperichondrium of the septum or the skin and perichondrium of the concha, a Negus suction dissector is invaluable.

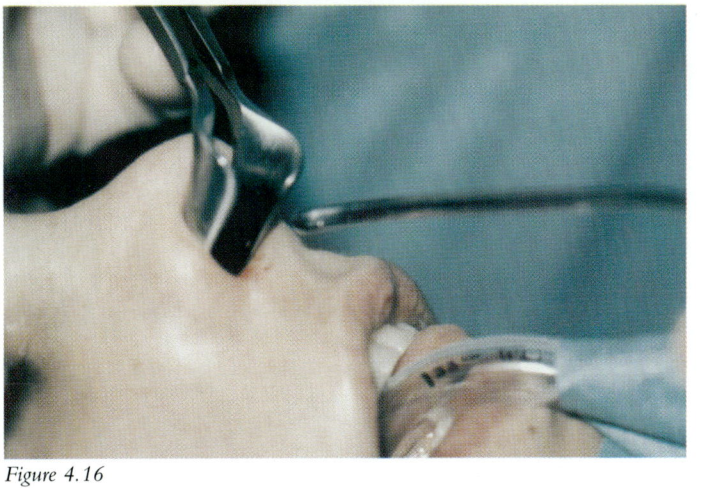

Figure 4.16

Incise the mucosa 1 cm from the caudal border. Insert a Negus dissector under the deepest layer of perichondrium, and strip off both surfaces of the septum by gentle side to side movements.

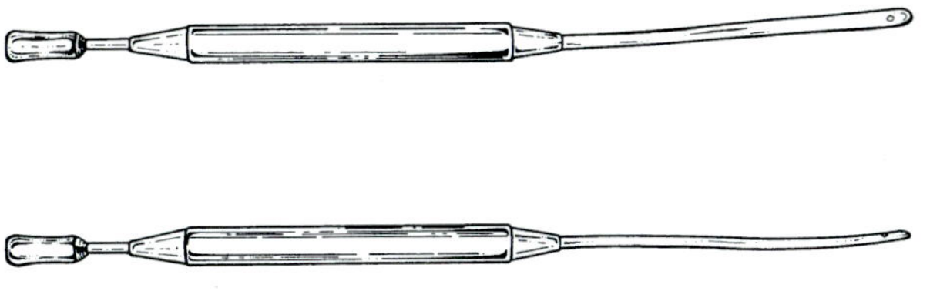

Figure 4.17

Then incise more deeply into the cartilage and strip off the mucoperichondrium on the other side with the same care.

Complete the dissection with a Ballanger swivel knife.

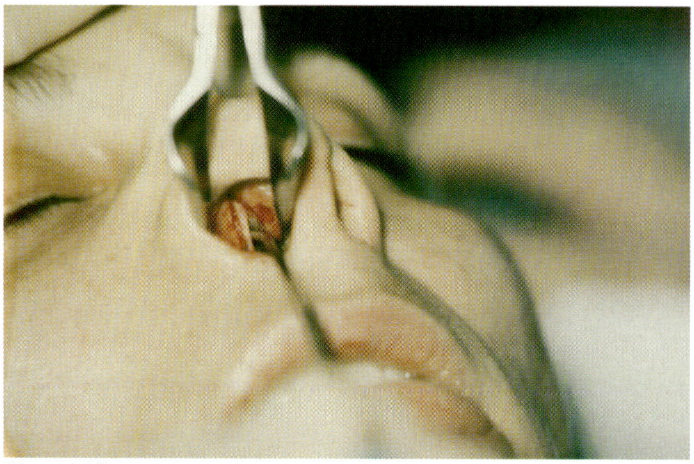
Figure 4.18

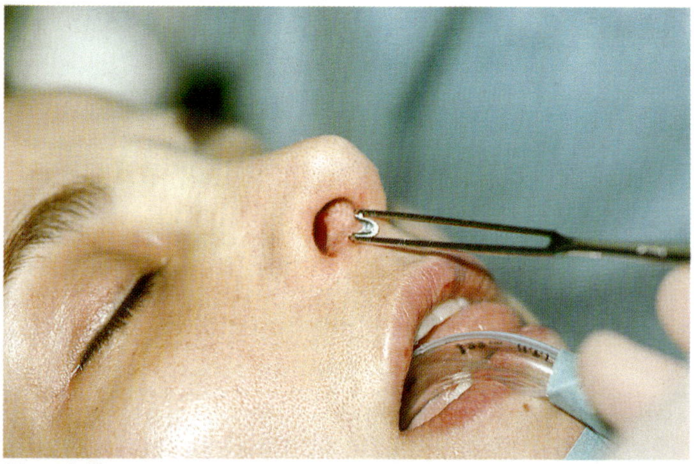
Figure 4.19

After removing the plate of septal cartilage, the thicker septal cartilage along the vomerine groove can be removed separately. This makes a good strut if needed for the columella.

Close the mucosa with a simple 4.0 plain catgut suture, leaving space for drainage.

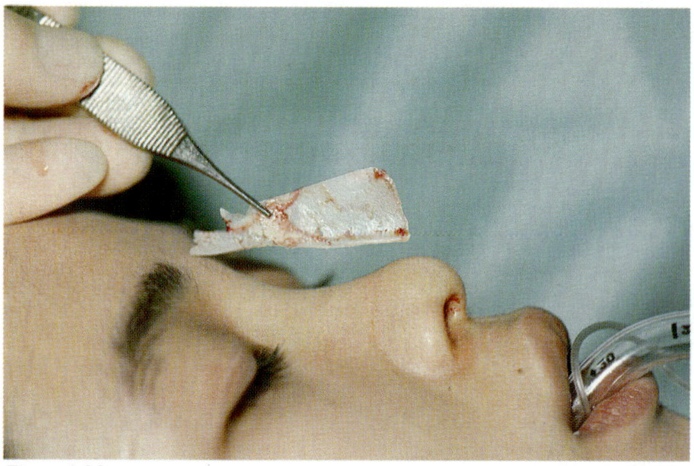
Figure 4.20

Concha

Obtain the conchal cartilage through an anterior incision just on the medial side of the antihelical fold. First inject the soft tissues with 1:200 000 adrenaline and then incise gently, extending the cut through the full thickness of the conchal cartilage.

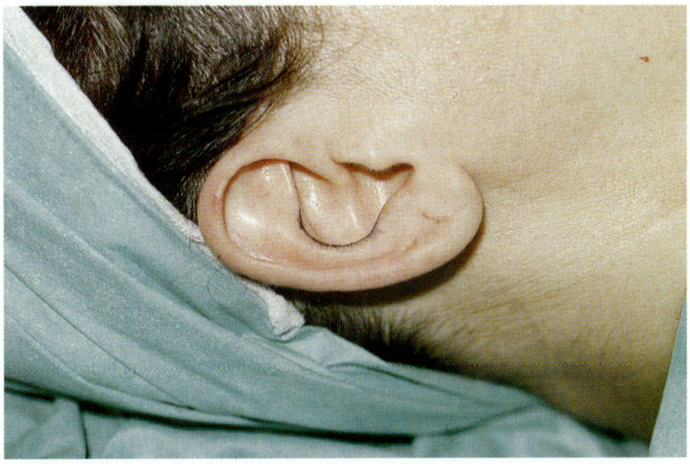

Figure 4.21

Strip the perichondrium carefully off the cartilage which is less adherent as the dissection advances into the depth of the concha.

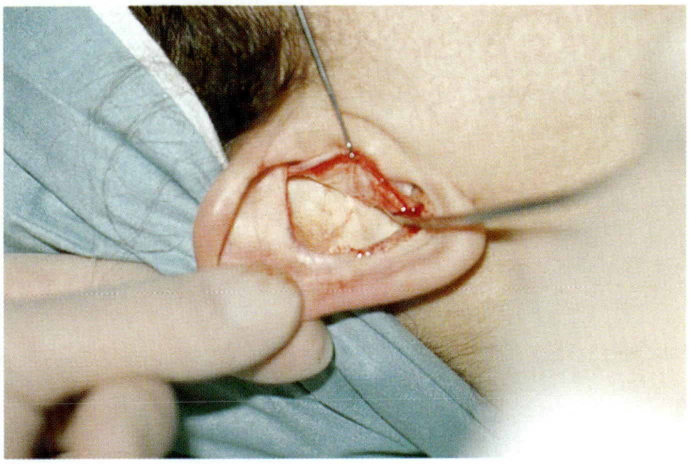

Figure 4.22

Carefully remove this cartilage in a single piece which usually measures up to 4.0 x 2.0 cm (Figure 4.24), giving adequate length for the dorsal nasal onlay.

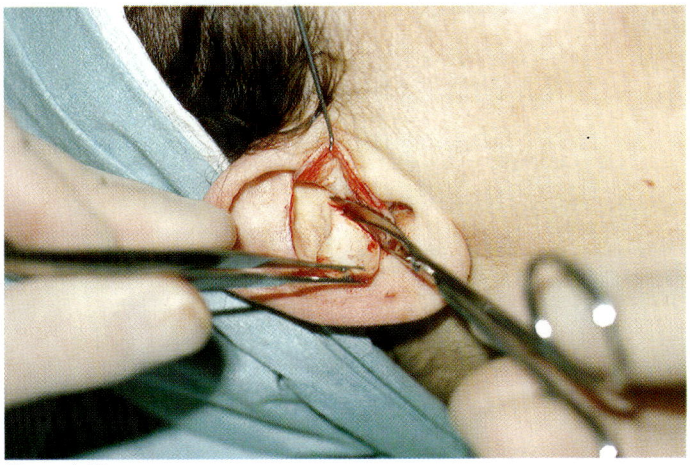

Figure 4.23

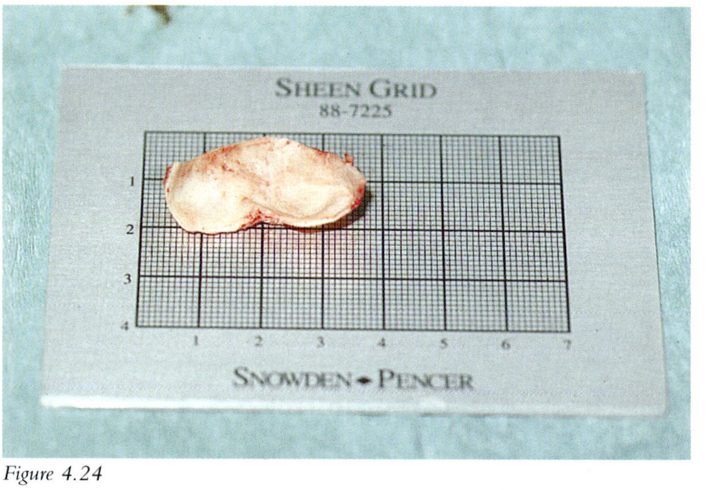

Figure 4.24

Leave these sutures long enough for securing a tie over dressing of cottonwool in the external canal and Sofratulle to fill out the concha.

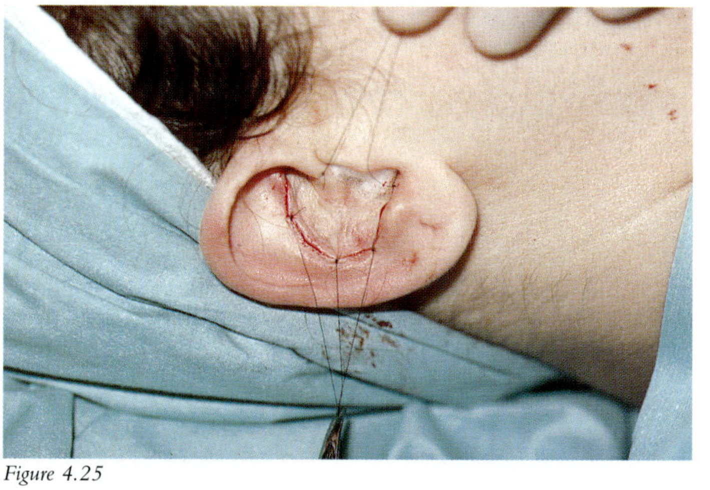

Figure 4.25

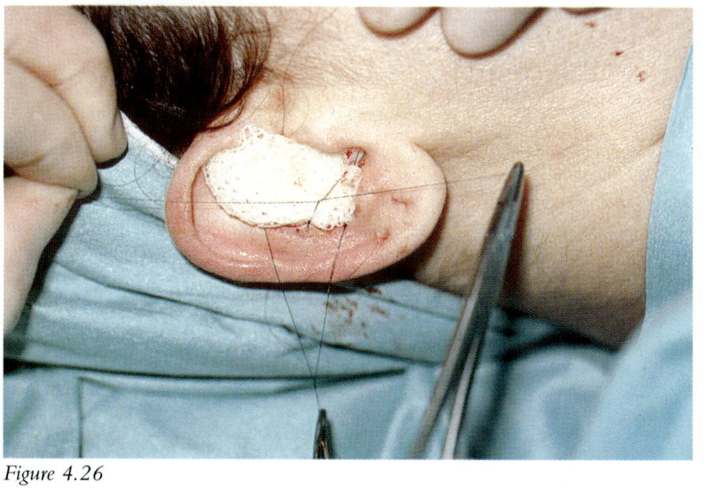

Figure 4.26

Complete this with a gauze dressing and 1 inch elastoplast. This avoids a cumbersome head bandage, is inconspicuous and much preferred by the patient.

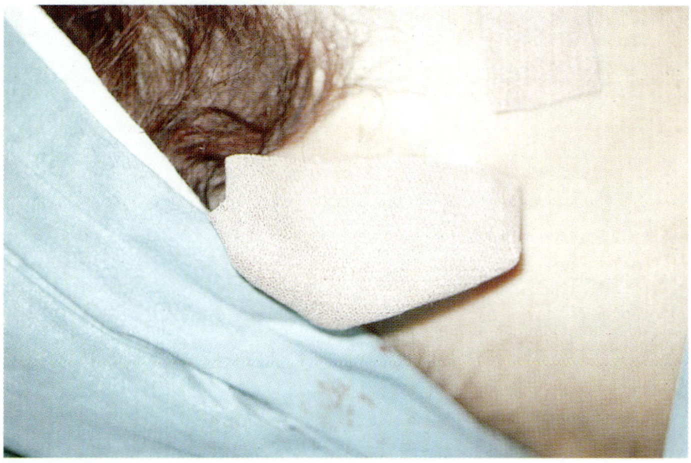

Figure 4.27

Carving and inserting the graft

Conchal grafts

The conchal graft measures approximately 3.5 x 2 cm. Cut a suitably sized piece from this, shave off the irregularities and bevel the edges.

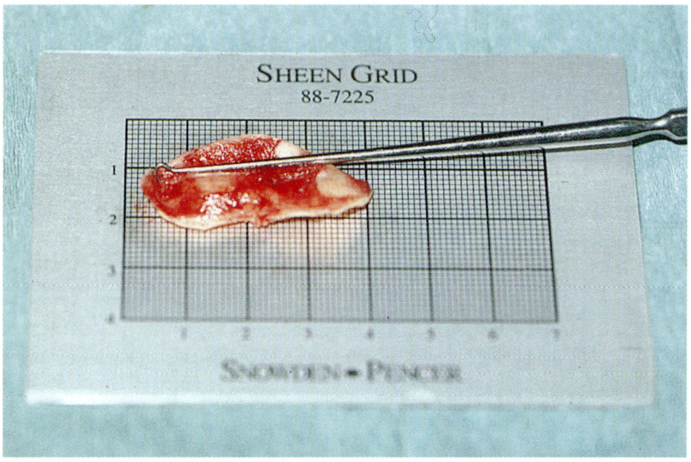

Figure 4.28

Flatten the graft further with a crusher.

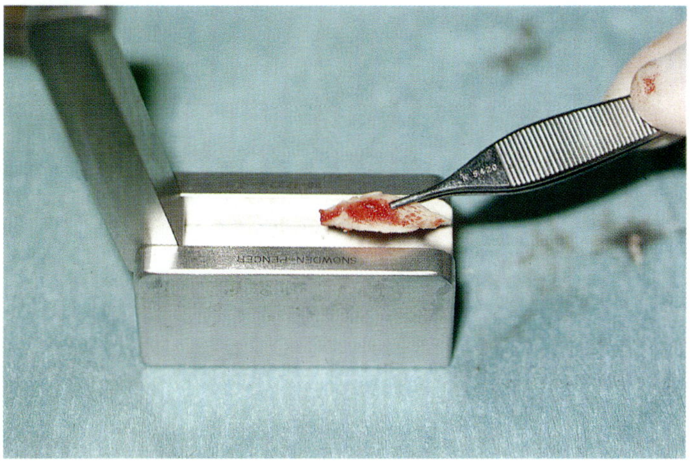

Figure 4.29

Flattened graft is now ready for insertion into the nose.

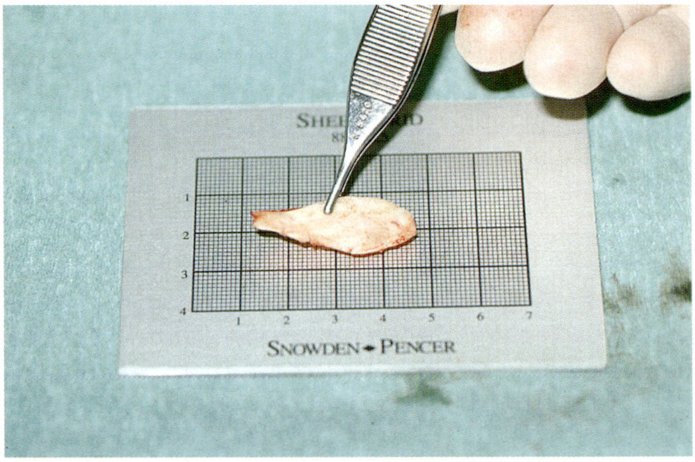

Figure 4.30

Introduce the graft into the dorsal pocket which is exposed by an Aufricht retractor.

When required, suture one or two additional layers on to the deep surface with fine catgut or collagen sutures.

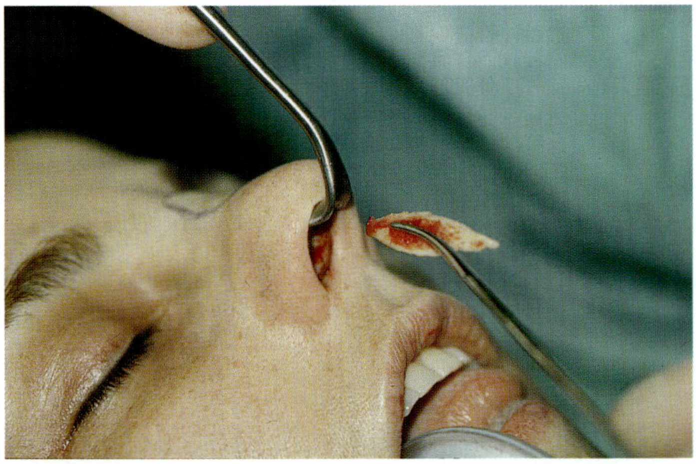

Figure 4.31

Septal grafts

The cartilage is more rigid and can be carved more precisely; consequently, it is superior for smooth onlay grafts to the supratip region of the dorsum. For larger dorsal grafts use the same technique as for conchal grafts, although scoring can be used to simulate dorsal convexity when required.

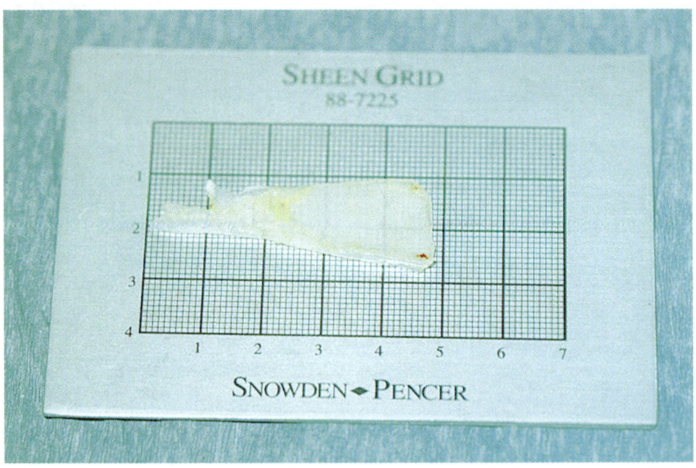

Figure 4.32

Additional columellar and tip grafts are introduced separately and according to individual requirements. The standard rhinoplasty dressing of Steristrips and Poroplast splint helps immobilize and protect the graft for 1 week postoperatively.

A gutter-shaped graft is formed by bevelling margins and parallel scoring of the convex side.

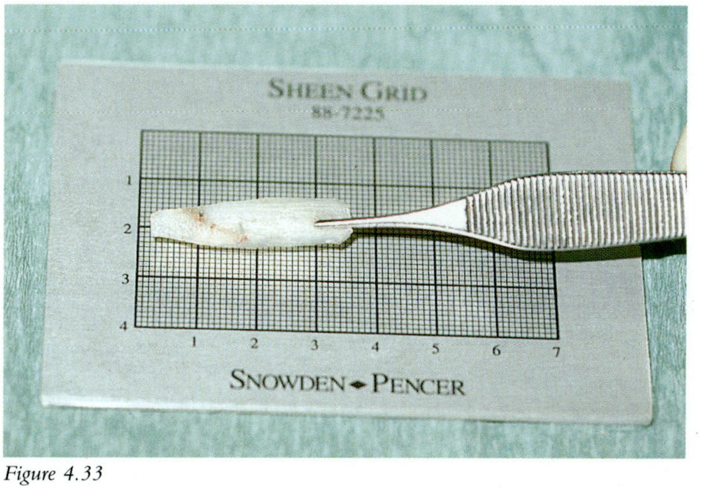

Figure 4.33

The pinched tip

Mechanisms of deformity

This results from a break in the spring of the tip cartilage supporting the nostril dome and nostril margin.

Division of the tip cartilage at this level must never be done unless the point of division is supported by an onlay tip graft, otherwise deformity will gradually occur, although often not apparent for a year or more.

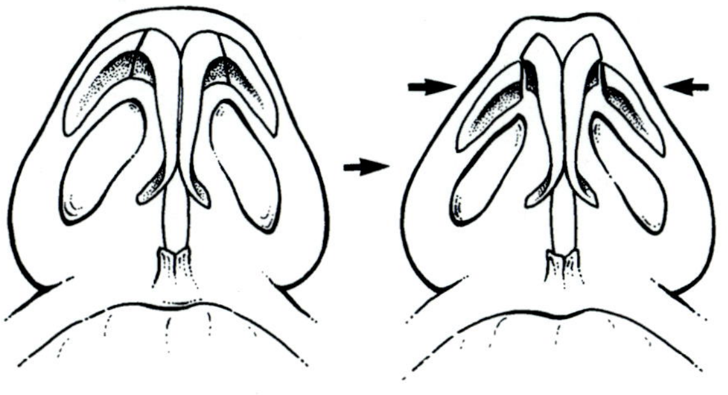

Figure 4.34

The most severe deformity of constricted tip will result when a segment of tip cartilage and nostril lining is excised from the nostril dome. With time the loss of the cartilaginous spring, first the scar tissue and later the forces of inspiration, will pull the cut ends of the lateral crura closer to the mid-line, forming a slit-like nostril and an unsightly constricted tip. Often the resultant deformity is asymmetrical as a result of a higher point on one of the cut ends of the medial crura.

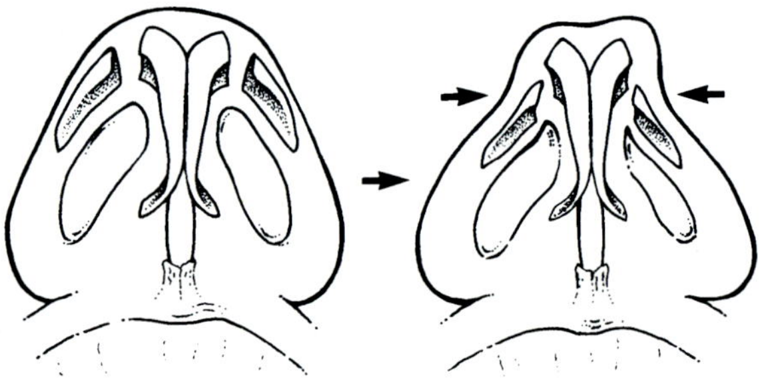

Figure 4.35a

Treatment

This is best done by trimming of the asymmetrical or excessive height of the medial crura and an onlay tip cartilage graft.

1. Expose the tip cartilages through a rim incision. If necessary further exposure can be obtained by intercartilaginous incision and bucket handle exposure of the cut ends of the tip cartilages. Additional incisions of this sort should be avoided if at all possible.
2. Excise the excessive prominence of the medial crura if this is deemed necessary; this then results in a lack of tip prominence and definition.

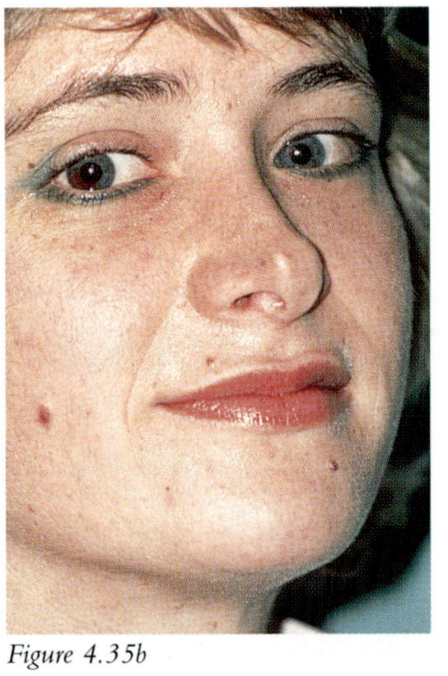

Figure 4.35b

In mild deformities An onlay tip graft carved from septal cartilage will restore the required tip prominence and shape as well as continuity of dome support.

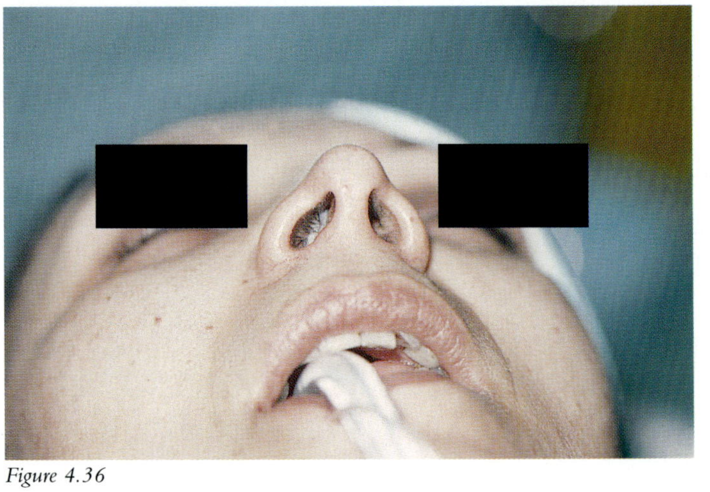

Figure 4.36

Design the size and shape of tip graft on the skin. A bilobed graft with finely tapering edges produces an attractive natural appearance. This may need to be heart shaped to fill a deficiency in the median crura. A second or even third layer of cartilage can be inserted deep to the first graft.

Undermine the skin cover in the mid-line of the tip sufficiently to accommodate the graft. The graft is now inserted and the nostril rim closed with 6.0 catgut sutures.

If the graft is found to be unstable, it is transfixed with 6.0 nylon which is brought out through the skin and loosely tied.

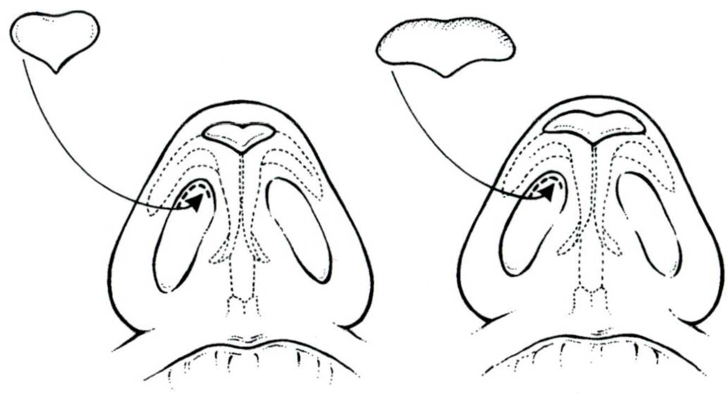

Figure 4.37

Immediately after a tip onlay graft.

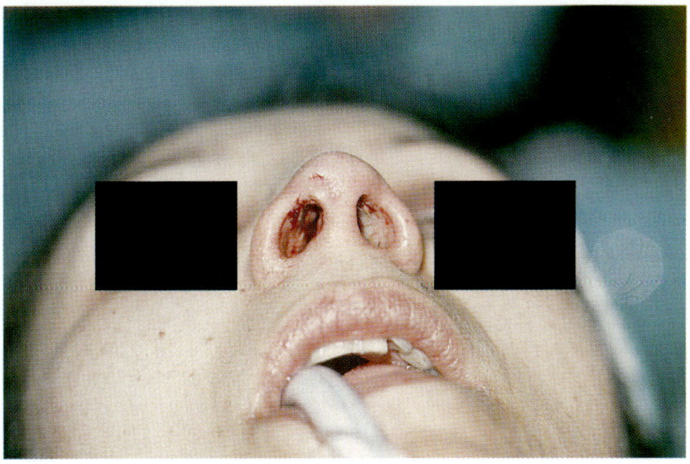

Figure 4.38

One year later: shape was maintained with appearance of normal attractive nasal tip or lobule.

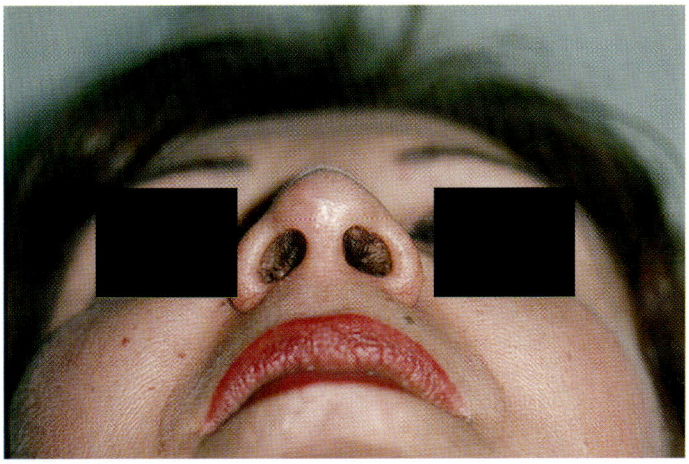

Figure 4.39

In severe deformities When the soft tissues are inelastic and scarred, gentle stretching will produce correction after which the graft is inserted.

A comma graft is preferred, because this adds a dynamic projection to the tip, as well as recreating the cartilaginous nostril domes. In such cases the soft tissue across the mid-line and the lobular portion of the tip are kept intact; the graft can therefore abut against the medial end of the pocket after insertion.

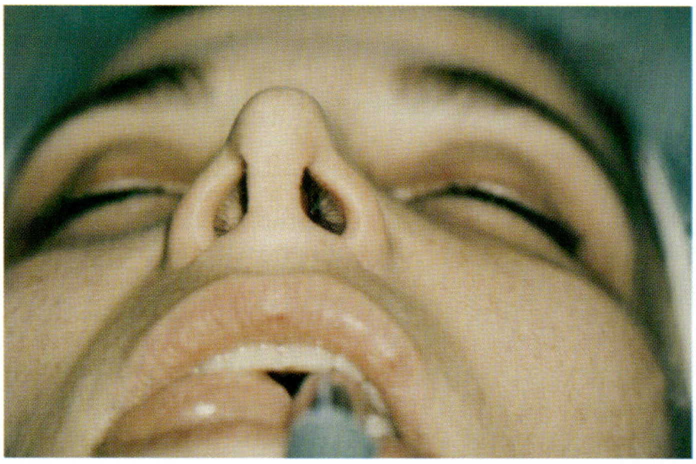

Figure 4.40

The subcutaneous pocket is carefully dissected allowing the pinched skin of the tip to expand. The dissection is extended along the nostril margin and superficial to the remaining lateral crus.

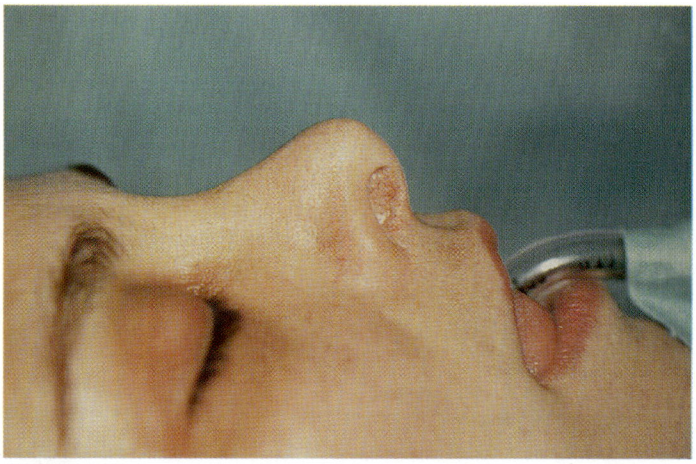

Figure 4.41

The graft is carved from septal cartilage whenever available because this can be finely bevelled to produce a flexible, springy structure with greater curve at the thinner medial end. The graft is up to 2 cm in length, and the medial end is curved to give the desired tip character and prominence. Insert the stiffer lateral end of the graft first.

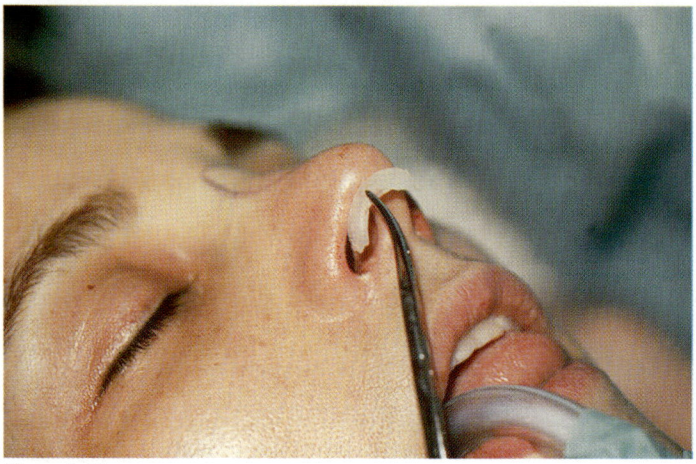

Figure 4.42

Apply traction with a skin hook to the skin incision near the tip and gently push the graft into the medial end of the pocket.
If too tight make increased space for the lateral end of the graft by gently undermining the skin with tip scissors.

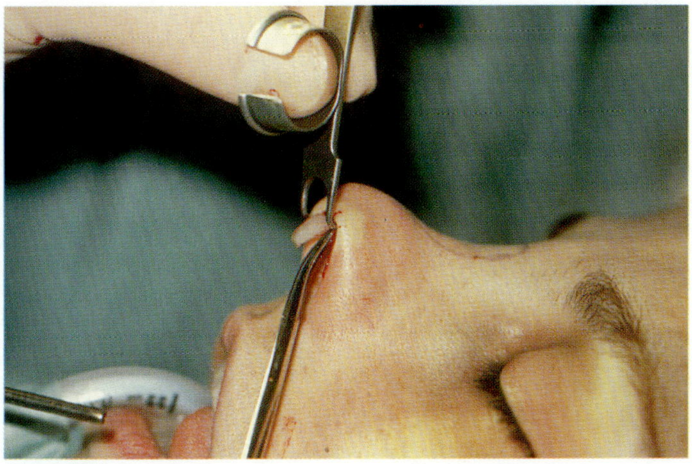

Figure 4.43

Before surgery the external valve is collapsed and narrowed.

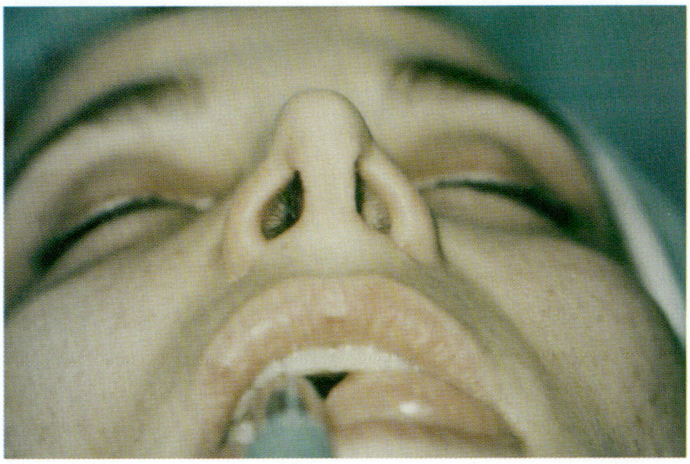

Figure 4.44

Now insert the graft on both sides and close the incisions with 6.0 catgut. The grafts should hold firmly in their pockets and produce immediately the desired correction of the tip deformity.
Note how this graft also achieves restoration of the external nasal valve.

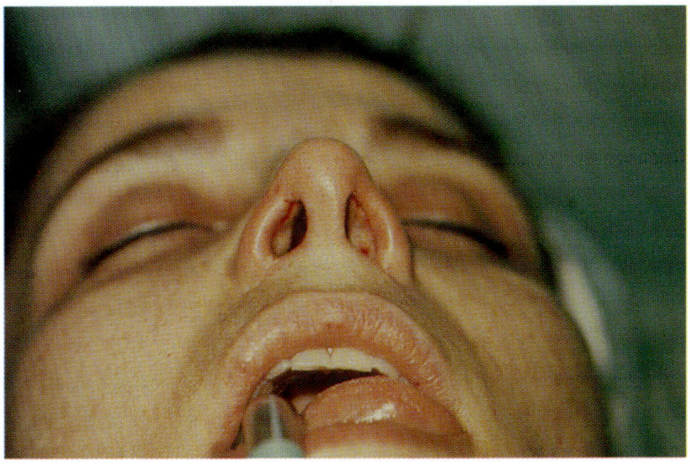

Figure 4.45

When the soft tissues are inelastic and scarred, gentle stretching will produce correction after which the graft is inserted more easily. Use the side and tips of the tip scissors to lift and stretch the soft tissues gently. Be patient and never exert more than gentle pressure.

Before surgery the tip is blunt and narrowed. Normal tip proportion is restored. A dorsal septal cartilage graft completes the procedure.

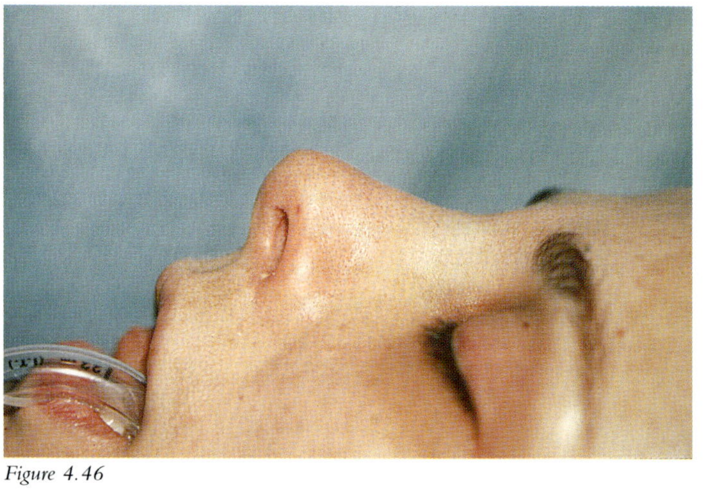

Figure 4.46

Clinical example

Another case of severe secondary deformity.

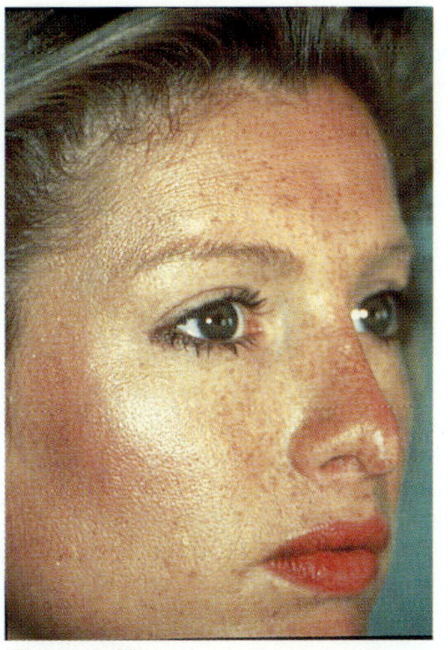

Figure 4.47

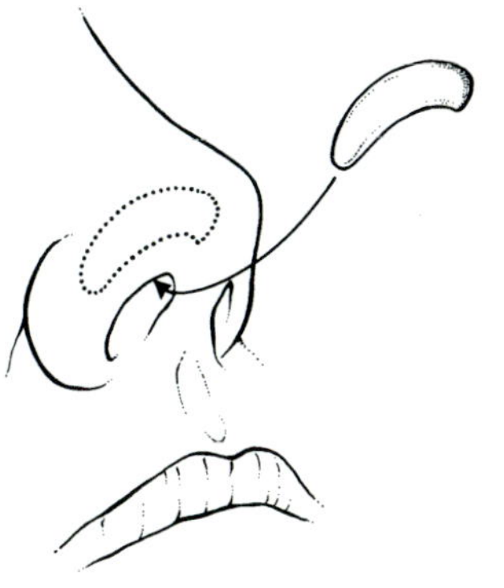

Figure 4.48

The comma graft is shaped with a bevelled medial end which then becomes both slightly bent and flexible.

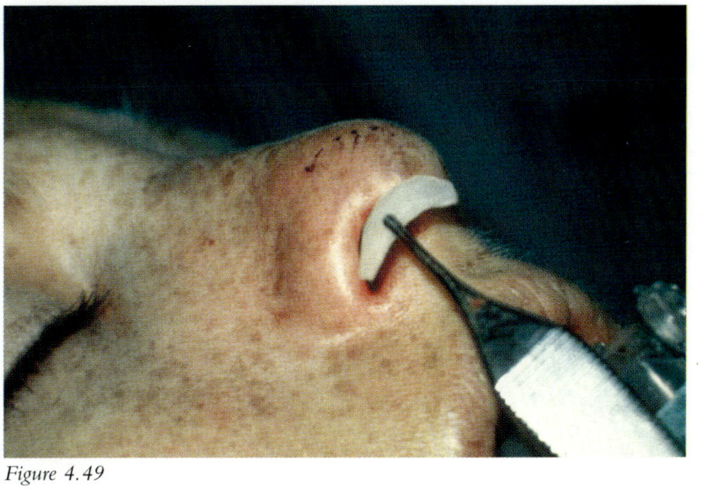

Figure 4.49

The result 7 years postoperatively, showing correction fully maintained.

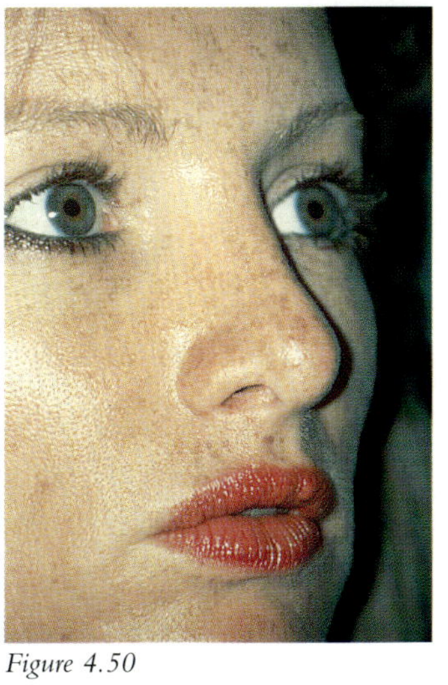

Figure 4.50

Clinical example

Pre- and 2 years postoperatively. External valve, and nasal tip reconstructions with comma grafts.

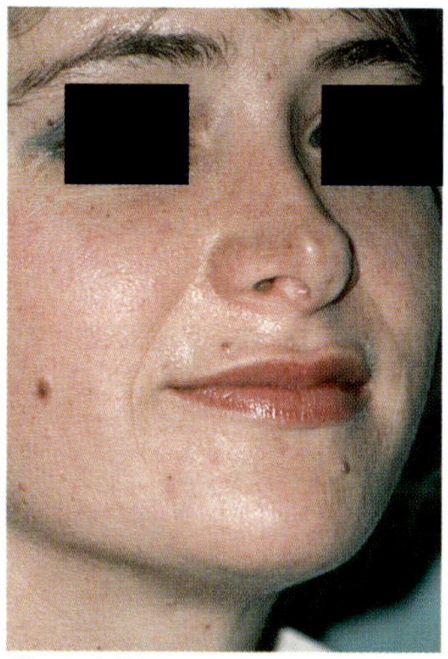

Figure 4.51a

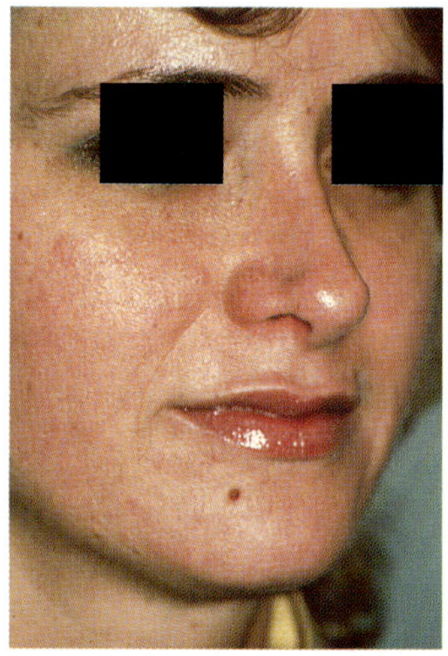

Figure 4.51b

Over-shortened nose with blunted tip.

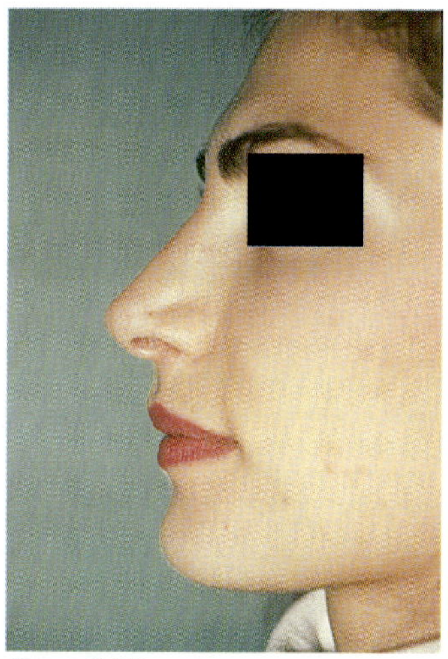

Figure 4.52

Intraoperative design for comma graft.

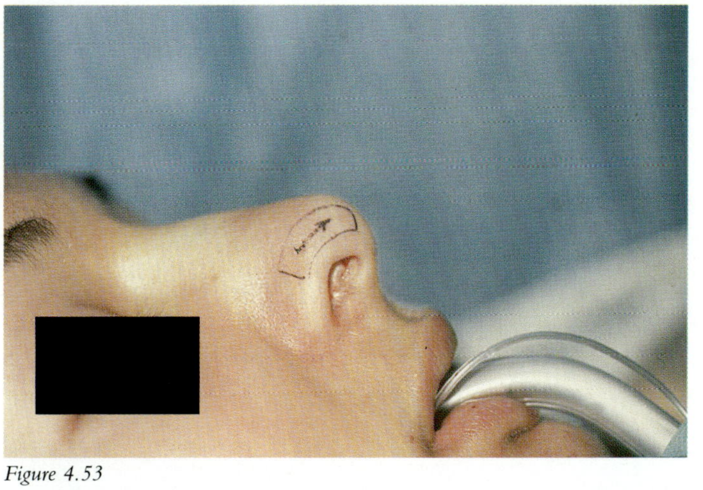

Figure 4.53

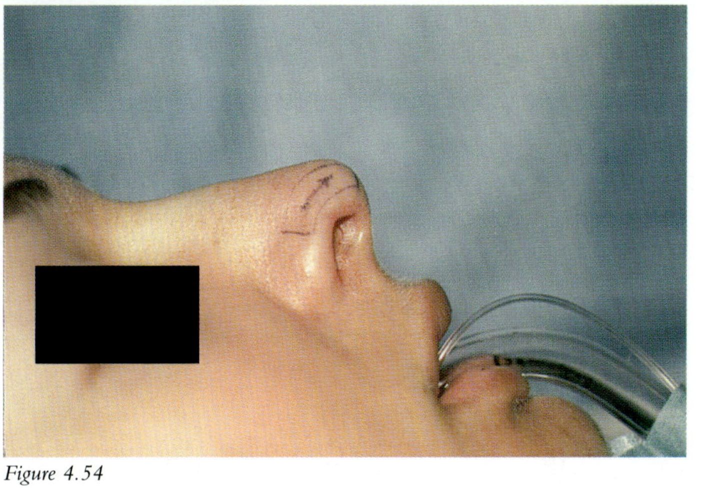

Figure 4.54

Appearance 1 year after surgery following comma graft to elongate nose and restore proper tip projection.

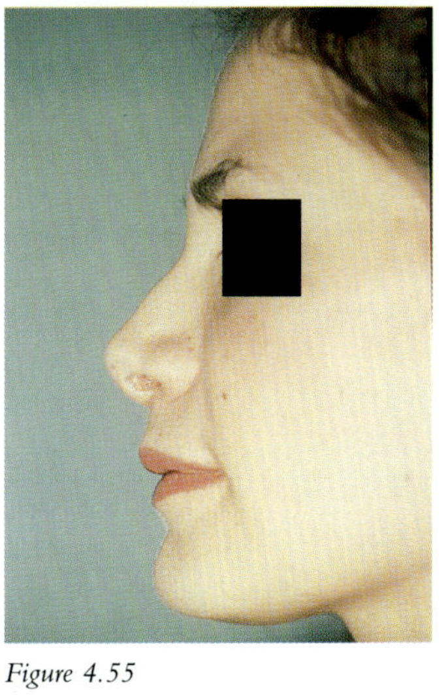

Figure 4.55

Supratip deformity

Supratip hump (or 'polly beak') deformity is a frequent post operative complication for the inexperienced surgeon.
There are three causes:

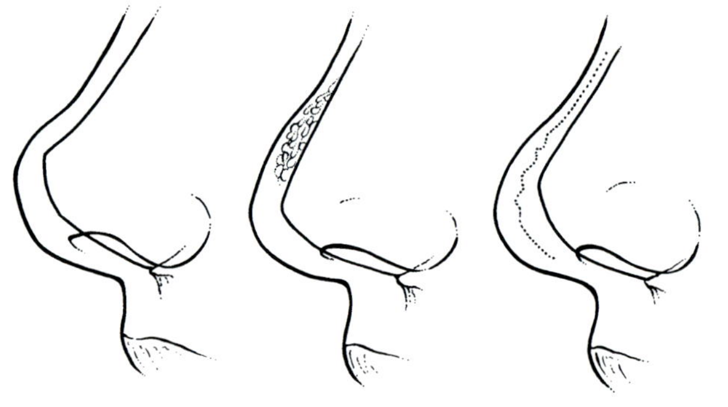

Figure 4.56

1. Inadequate lowering of the dorsal hump or accidental neglect of a septal spur produces a septal hump. This is palpable and becomes more apparent when the patient smiles. It often becomes more apparent after a few months when the tip has dropped a little, and the soft tissues and skin have softened.
Reoperate after 6 months and lower the septum to a correct level.

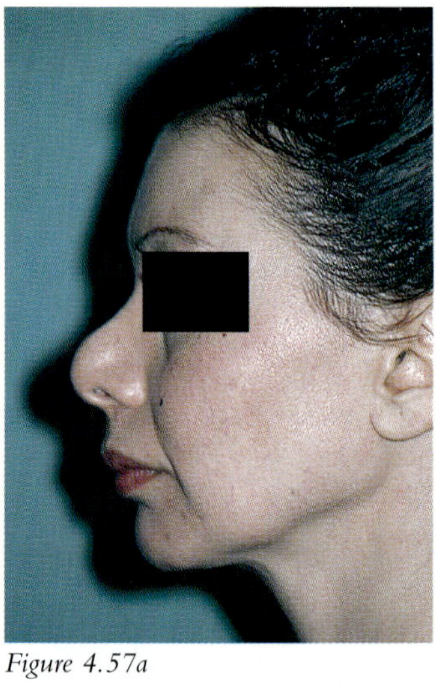

Figure 4.57a

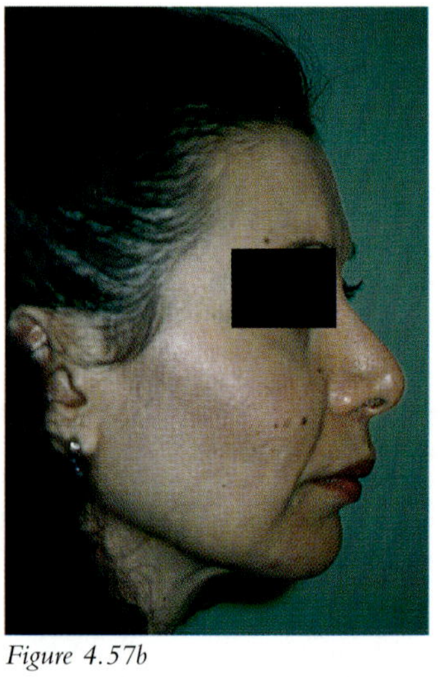

Figure 4.57b

2. A wide tip or bulbous tip with thick sebaceous skin will often have an important amount of underlying fibrofatty tissue. If left, this will cause a soft rubbery supratip swelling. This basic step is already described (see page 28).
Undermine the soft tissues of the dorsum to allow re-draping of the skin, and remove the excess fibrofatty tissue under the supratip skin or attached to the cartilaginous dorsum.

3. Over-reduction of the cartilaginous skeleton in a wide nose may result in a supratip hump. This occurs if the overlying skin is too thick and inelastic to be able to shrink down and accommodate to the smaller size.
To correct this deformity the skeleton must be subtly enlarged, usually by means of a tip cartilage graft and dorsal onlay graft. A short columella is a secondary contributing factor, and therefore an umbrella graft or columellar strut will be required in such a situation.

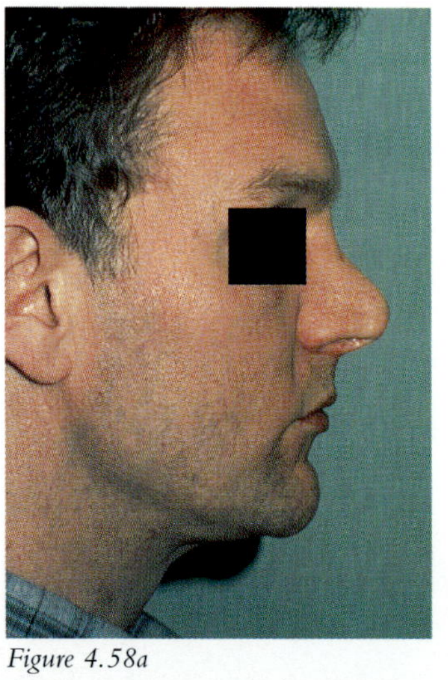

Figure 4.58a

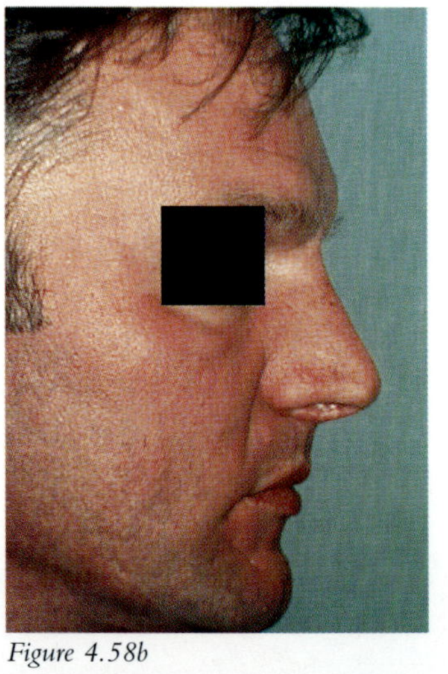

Figure 4.58b

Part V

Ethnic Characteristics and Aesthetic Harmony

Ethnic Characteristics and Aesthetic Harmony

In the past much emphasis has been placed on *reduction rhinoplasty* which traditionally implied 'removal of the bony hump and infracture, narrowing and refinement of the nasal tip'.

Fortunately our standards have not only much increased with a greatly increased trend to augmentation rhinoplasty, but we now also recognize the varying objectives for differing sexes, facial character and ethnic types.

Rhinoplasty of the male

Trauma is a more frequently associated factor, so that nasal obstruction is often the major complaint. The patient may ask to have his nose restored to the original shape, as well as correcting the nasal airway obstruction.

Others will see this as an opportunity to improve their appearance — to obtain less of the 'prize fighter's' nose and a more photogenic look.

Those patients who do not have any history of post-traumatic deformity may frequently express a desire to improve on their hereditary large nose and for this treatment is straightforward.

There are, among this group, patients who display a perfectionist tendency or an underlying obsession, and with these patients great care must be taken.

In all these groups there is therefore a varying but also a substantial reason for greater conservatism than in rhinoplasty in the average female.

Just as with blepharoplasty or face lift in the males care must be taken not to over-treat because this will create a bland or effeminate appearance.

The patient may see this not only as a failure of the rhinoplasty, but as if his character has been taken away. This will then lead to patient dissatisfaction, resentment and possible litigation.

When post-traumatic deformity and dysfunction exist, make this the primary objective of the operation.

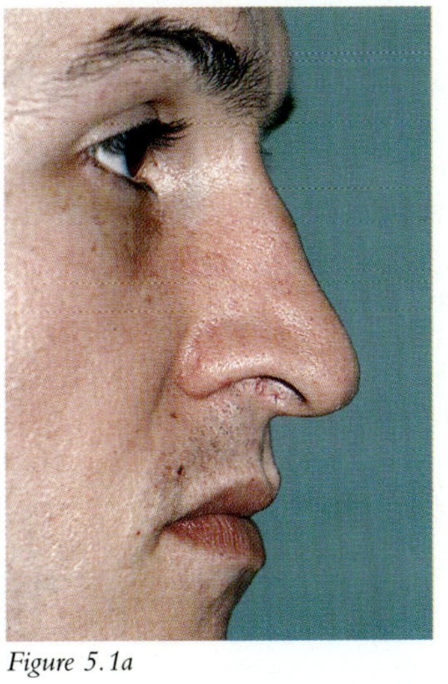

Figure 5.1a

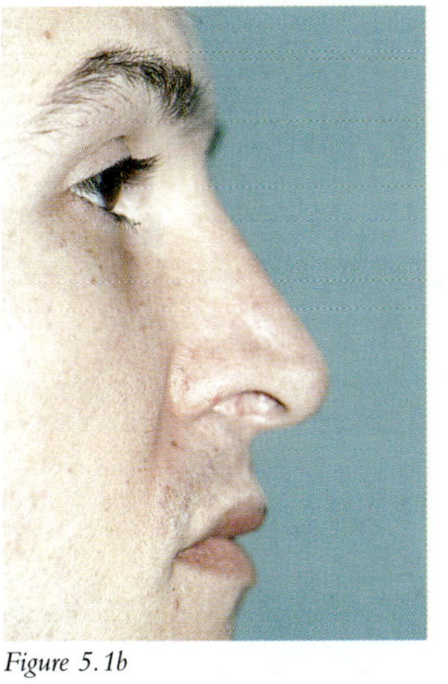

Figure 5.1b

Correction of external deformities

Restoration of symmetry

This is a frequent requirement. Long-standing deformity from childhood injury is usually impossible to correct fully because of soft tissue asymmetry, and the tendency to 'creep' back to the original shape. An onlay dorsal graft will often succeed in masking this type of deformity.

Post-traumatic hump

The male nose characteristically has a more barrel-shaped bony dorsum and mild hump. These features should be preserved and a clear objective established with the patient. Rasping down of an excessive hump may be all that is necessary.

Retracted columella

This is a frequent finding in association with deviated nasal septum.

In such cases, a photographic record of the patient's profile, smiling as well as in repose, is useful.

Insert a T-shaped columellar maxillary strut as illustrated on page 78. Frequently two or three struts will be required, carved from the septal cartilage.

Hanging tip

Excessive length of the nose or hanging tip may be associated with a retracted columella. Treatment is described on page 64.

Refinement of the nasal tip

The nasal tip of the male is not only larger but characteristically less delicate in appearance; the tip cartilages produce a rounder tip with greater differentiation from the dorsum. The nose is longer with a more acute columellar-labial angle of 90°.

Never over-refine the tip cartilages or over-shorten the nose. Be conservative and do not be persuaded to carry out requests that are against your instinctive judgement.

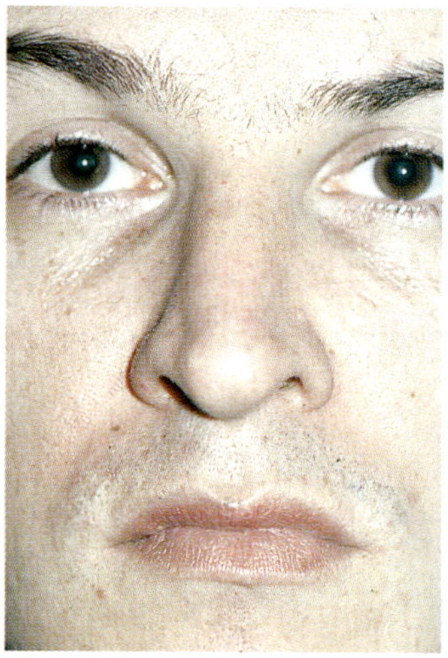

Figure 5.2a

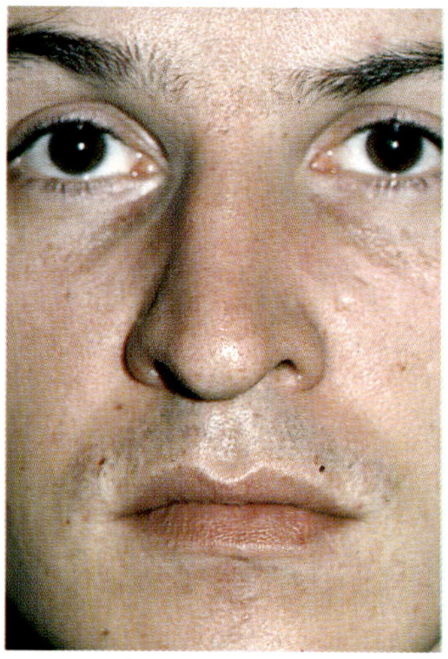

Figure 5.2b

The ageing nose

Introduction

The adult nose changes with age, and, is well illustrated in many artists studies, in particular those of Leonardo da Vinci.

Relaxation of the connective tissues causes the nose to elongate and the tip to drop.

The skin will often become coarser, contributing to enlargement of the tip and thickening of the nostrils. In some cases the tip cartilages appear to enlarge making the tip more bulbous and the nostrils more flared.

Assessment

Be conservative. The objective is to create harmony as well as a degree of rejuvenation. Over-shortening or over-reduction in the nose can create contradiction in an otherwise more mature and dignified appearance.

If well performed, a conservative rhinoplasty can enhance a facelift and give harmony of appearance.

Treatment

Rhinoplasty may conveniently be performed at the time of a facelift, provided that a reasonably conservative and straightforward operation is anticipated. Otherwise it is wiser to postpone and perform rhinoplasty at a second stage.

The treatment plan will usually consist of the following:

1. Conservative refinement of the tip cartilages.
2. Shortening of the relaxed membranous portion of the nasal septum.
3. Conservative hump reduction and infracture.

When performed alone, a full rhinoplasty may be carried out as for a younger patient. The skeletal tissues handle differently. Beware of the often harder and more brittle bones and take greater care with the infracture.

Remember that the less elastic older skin will not adapt as readily.

The tip cartilages are more friable and are

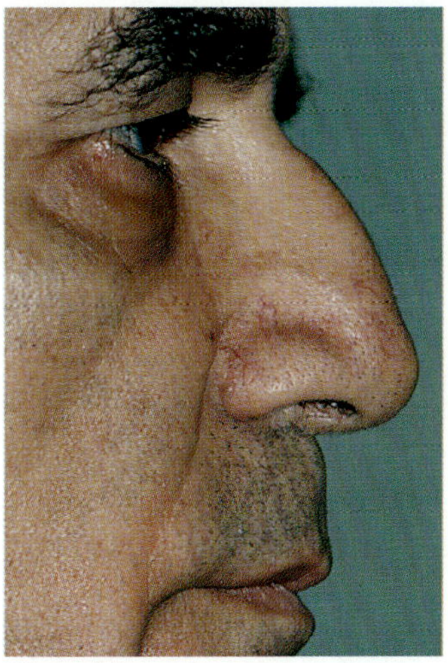

Figure 5.3a

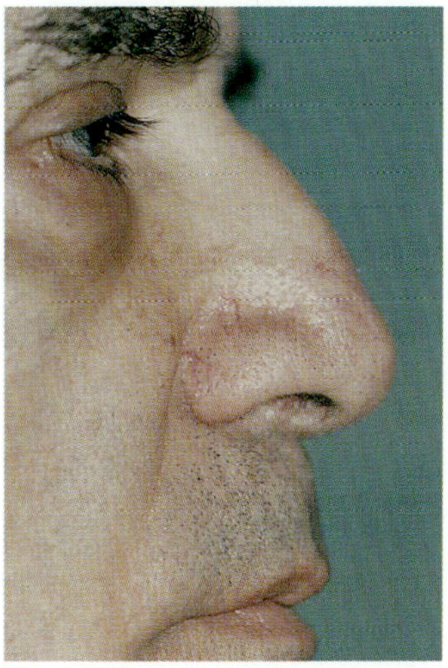

Figure 5.3b

easily torn; therefore dissection must be done with added caution.

Ethnic variations

Within this chapter it is only possible to pick out the most obvious examples of ethnic difference, which can serve as the basis for more detailed study. But even this is sufficient to highlight the most important aspects of our appreciation and understanding in designing the appropriate nasal modifications of an individual's nose.

The oriental nose

This is characterized by a short low dorsum, a round wide nasal tip and a short columella with an acute columellar-labial angle.

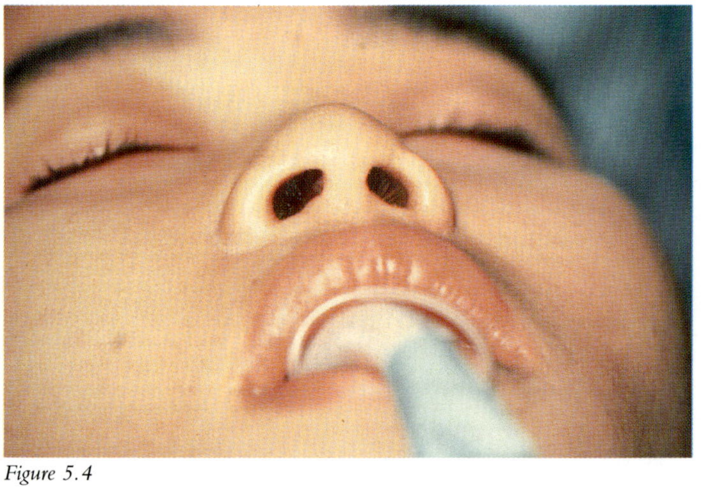

Figure 5.4

The columella frequently projects forward with convex shape.

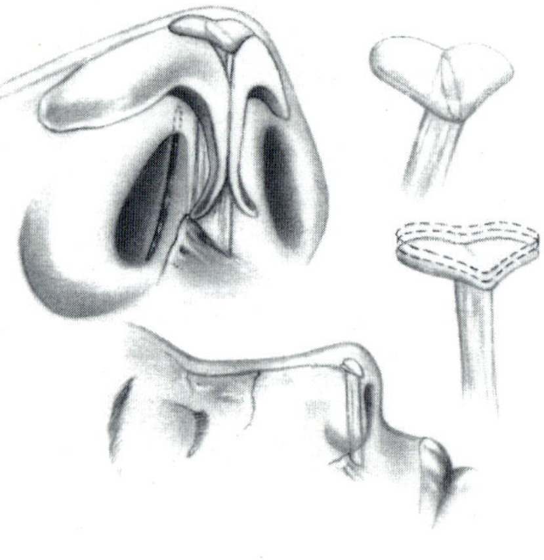

Figure 5.5

Requests for dorsal augmentation are common, not only for aesthetic reasons but also so that sunglasses can be worn without slipping.

Dorsal augmentation
I prefer to use an onlay of up to three layers of septal cartilage, but if this is not adequate a aloplastic material may be unavoidable (page 90).

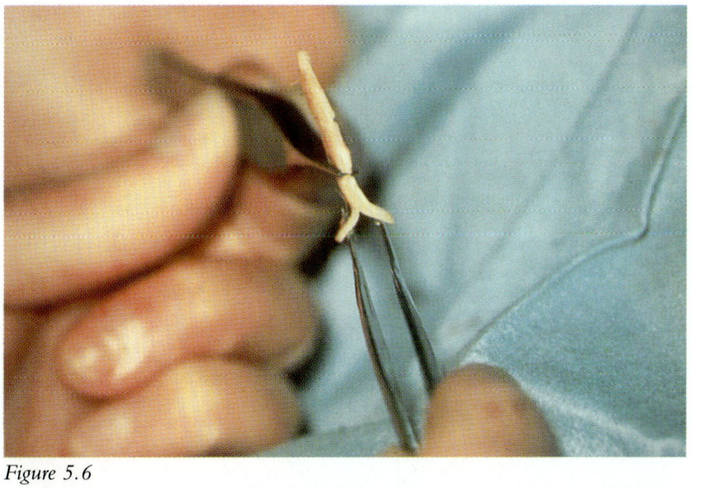
Figure 5.6

Tip augmentation with an umbrella graft is the preferred method (see page 80). The tip grafts are an essential part and give refinement to the tip. These alterations produce a harmonious effect and enhance the overall facial appearance.

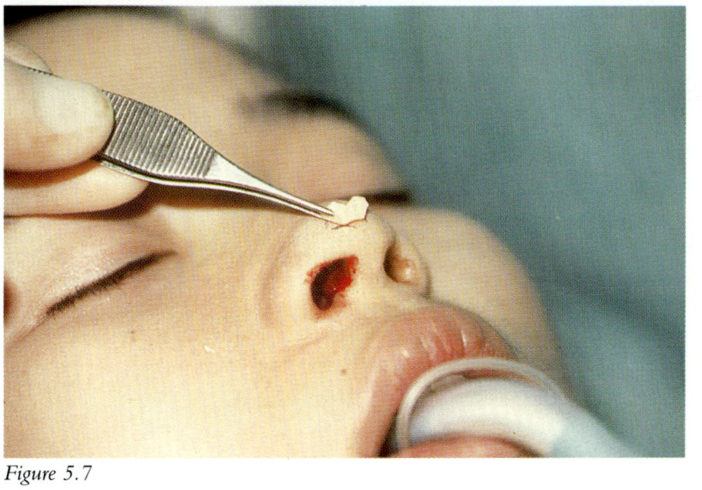
Figure 5.7

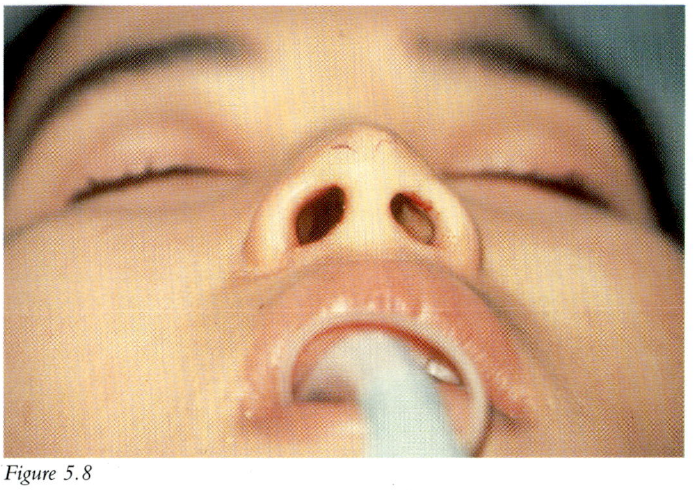
Figure 5.8

The Indian nose

The type of nose seeking rhinoplasty is most frequently characterised by:

1. Broad dorsum
2. High septal dorsum
3. Broad tip cartilages.

This nose is quite easily corrected by reduction of the appropriate structures, but avoid excessive reduction, because the mouth and upper lip are of generous size with full vermilion.

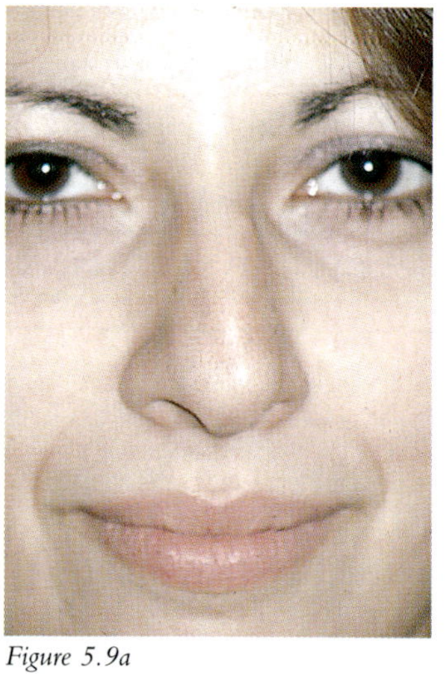

Figure 5.9a

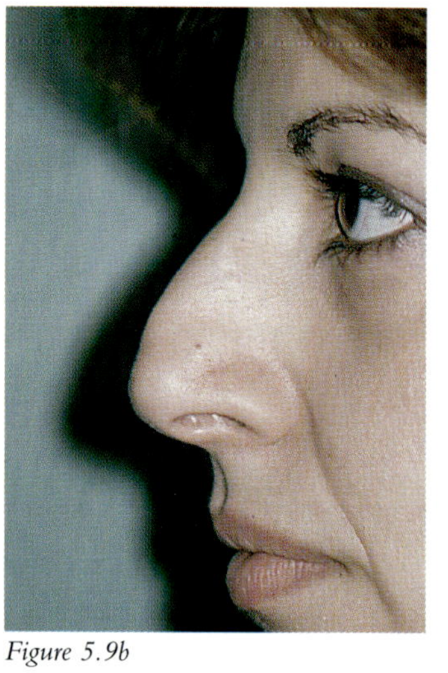

Figure 5.9b

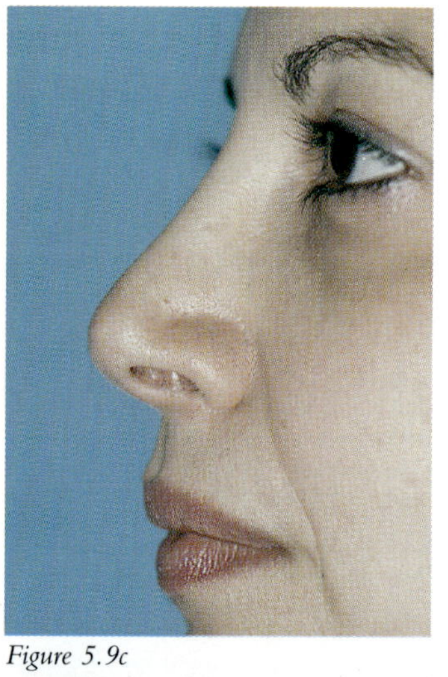

Figure 5.9c

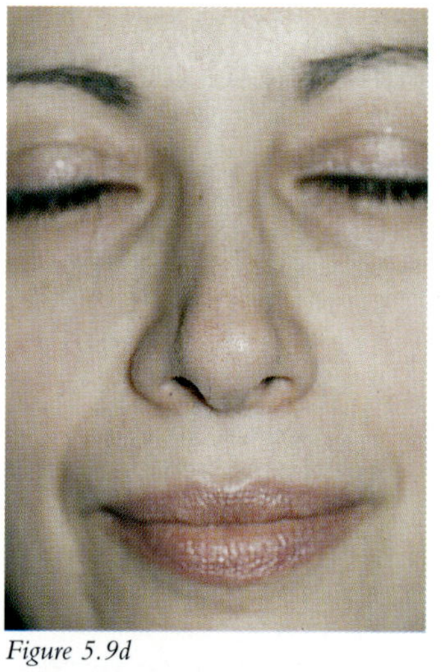

Figure 5.9d

Another example

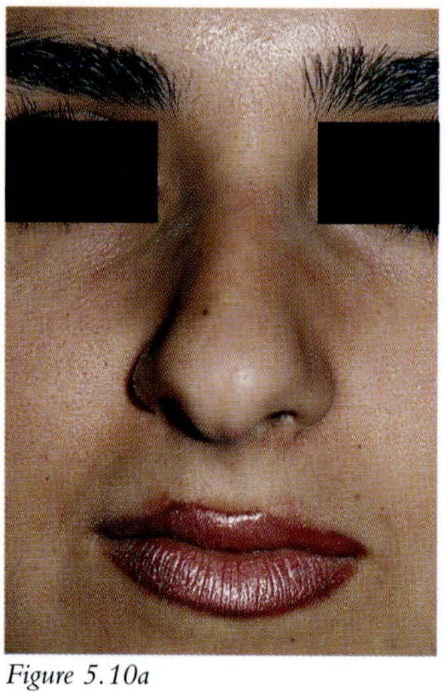

Figure 5.10a

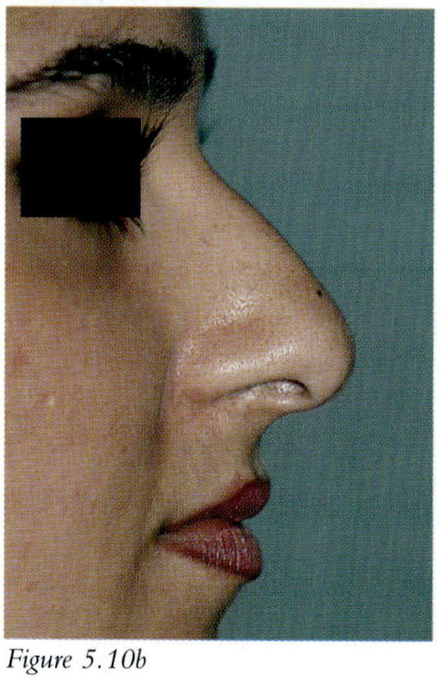

Figure 5.10b

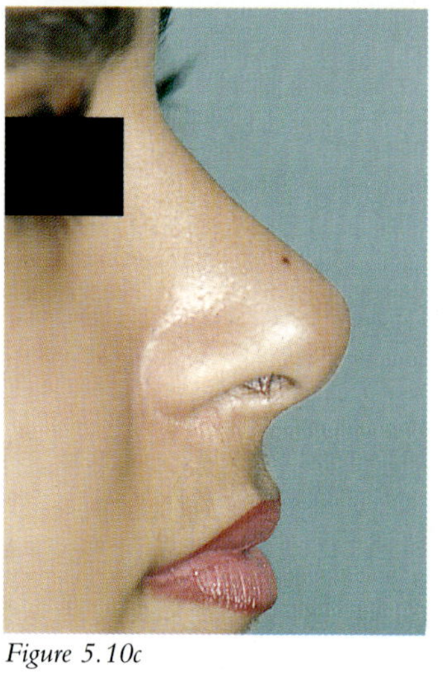

Figure 5.10c

The negroid nose

There is considerable variation among Afro-Caribbean people, but the outstanding characteristics of the stereotypical nose are made up of a low wide bony profile, and a blunt tip with wide nostrils and sebaceous skin.

The dorsal height may be sufficient and cannot be altered without disturbing the overall facial harmony, which is sometimes seen with the characteristic backward sloping forehead and wide lips.

Elevation of the tip and appropriate tip refinement (in the female) can best be achieved with an umbrella graft (see page 80).

Wide nostrils

These may result from a wide nostril floor. Remove an oblique wedge immediately medial to the nostril base.

Mark the planned elliptical excision with maximum width at the nostril sill. Design this incision to run obliquely downwards and laterally, because this will prevent notching of the scar at the nostril sill.

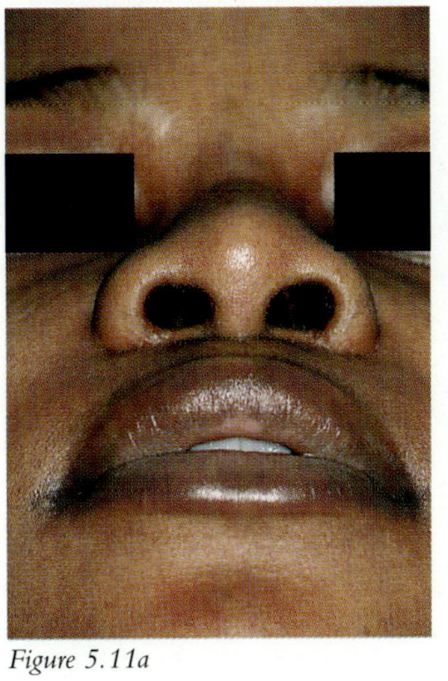

Figure 5.11a

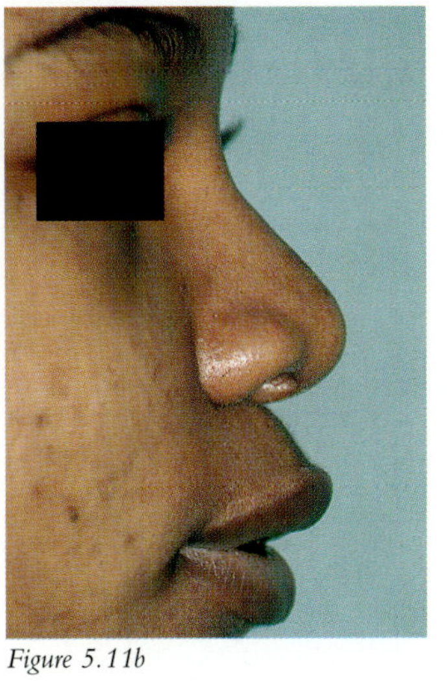

Figure 5.11b

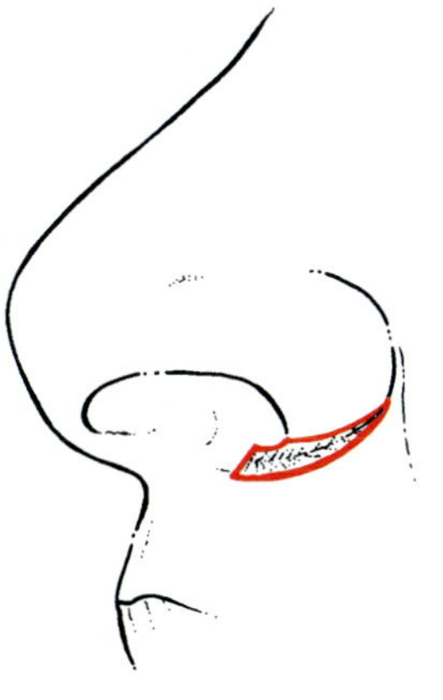

Figure 5.12a

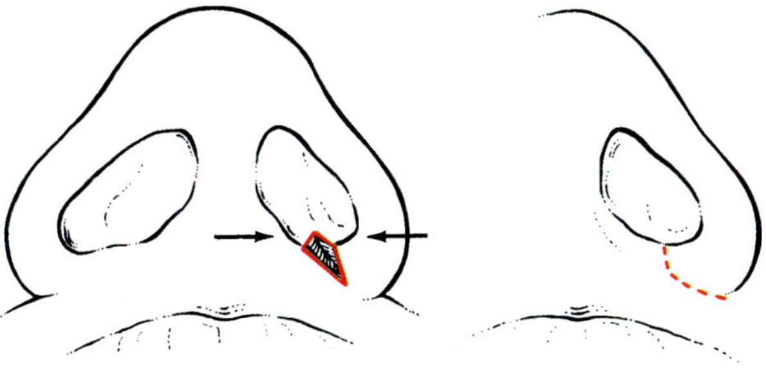

Figure 5.12b

Close the incision with a 4.0 catgut suture subcutaneously in the nostril floor, and three to four interrupted 6.0 nylon skin sutures.
The nose then has improved aesthetic harmony without loss of ethnic character. Sometimes the nostrils are large and also flared and will require wedge excision at the base. Always keep the external incision to a minimum.
Debulking of wide alae is done classically by external elliptical skin excision, which produces an undesirable visible scar in the sebaceous thick skin.

Instead a similar effect can be produced by an internal approach.
Incise the inner nasal skin superficially for a 1 cm length directly opposite the part of the alae to be reduced.
Excise an ellipse of subcutaneous tissue to the full thickness of the alae.
Close the incision with two or three interrupted 4.0 catgut sutures, including a little of the soft tissue remaining at the depth of the excision.

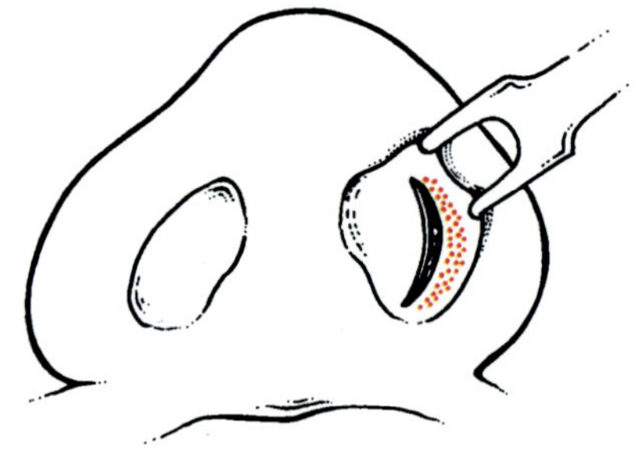

Figure 5.13

Excision of the alar base

In some cases the apparently wide nostril base will in reality result from flared nostrils. A suitably designed wedge excision from the nostril base is then required.
Mark the proposed skin excision at the alar crease.
Maximum width of excision is at the nostril rim, tapering appropriately laterally and medially.
Do not attempt to be too radical because this will distort the final result. Wide nostrils are a natural characteristic and should be kept in harmony with the relatively blunt nasal tip, full lips and generous mouth.

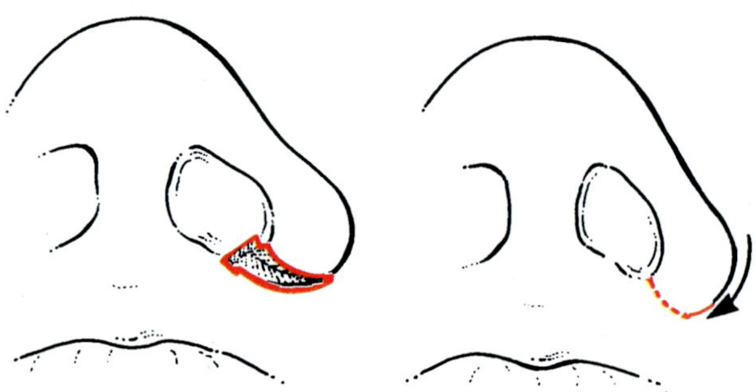

Figure 5.14

The Jewish nose

This is frequently characterized by a high narrow aquiline bony and cartilaginous dorsum, and broader hanging tip.

Others may have an altogether wider nose with thick sebaceous skin and rounded tip. Correction requires a classic rhinoplasty with lowering of the dorsum, narrowing of the bony pyramid, refinement and elevation of the excessively long hanging tip. Tip projection is usually pronounced requiring reduction rather than augmentation.

The Middle Eastern or North African nose

There are many variations, although characteristically the nose is long with hanging tip. This is also a frequent characteristic in Spanish features and was produced by the Moorish influence.

The 'bottom heavy' quality may frequently pose problems. Treatment requires judgement between build-up of the radix of the nose and reduction of the cartilaginous dorsum. If the columella is short, special caution is required or a secondary polly-beak deformity will result.

After appropriate shortening and refinement of the dorsum and tip, use the redundant dorsal cartilage as a crushed cartilage graft to the radix.

Take septal cartilage and use this for a multi-layered columellar T graft to augment the columella and anterior maxilla.

Only in exceptional cases will a tip graft also be required, because the shortened anterior third of the septum will give the tip upward rotation and sufficient projection.

The European Nose

In spite of ever increasing cross-breeding, there are still striking national characteristics that influence the choice of rhinoplasty design.

The *northern European* nose of the Nordic type represents an 'ideal' form being characteristically straight with small well sculpted tip cartilages. The facial character is also well proportioned, with fair skin and blonde straight hair and long head. The German features tend to be heavier features with a broader and larger nose.

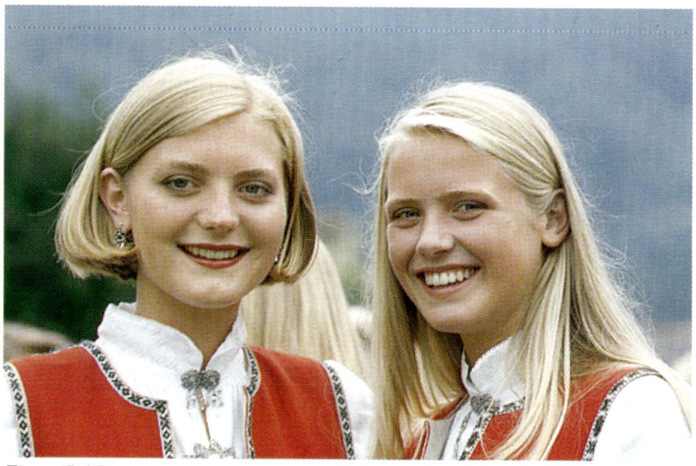

Figure 5.15

In western Europe there are still remnants of the Celtic race with red-hair, freckled skin and a short straight nose that is somewhat similar to the nose of the Nordic peoples; usually, however, the nose is a little more upturned and broader tipped — one that is youthful in appearance.

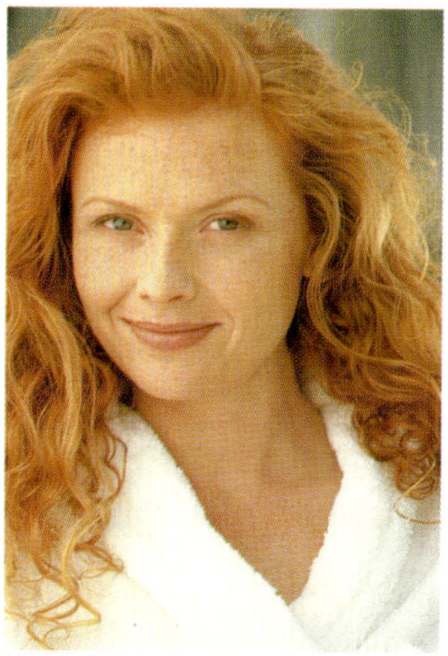

Figure 5.16

The *eastern European* or Slavonic races have a straight nose, although it is often larger and the eyes are more closely approximated.

The Alpine races have similar characteristics, with darker hair, closer set eyes and a narrower longer nose.

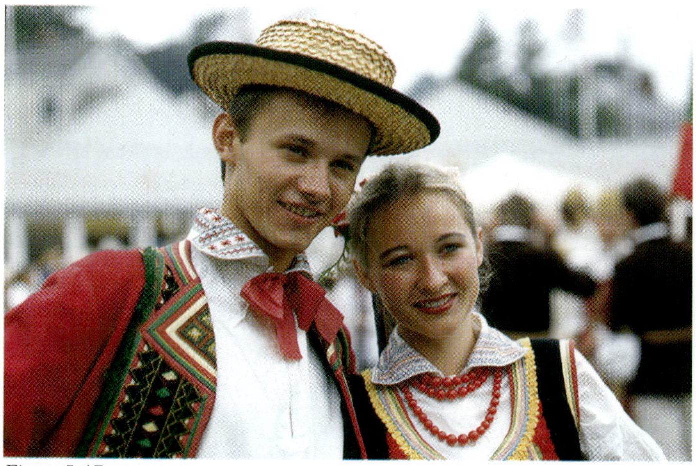

Figure 5.17

The *southern European* or Mediterranean races are characteristically of shorter build with round heads and darker straight hair. The nose is long and aquiline, although it is broader in the peoples from more eastern Mediterranean countries.

Italians have finer features with wider set eyes and generous lips.

Spaniards provide a more complex and mixed race, although the Moorish influence gives a longer nose of markedly aquiline character and often a smallish chin with narrower lips and a longer head than the Italian.

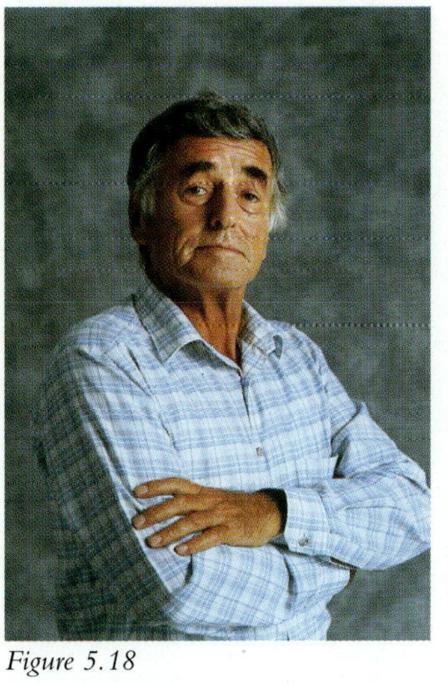

Figure 5.18

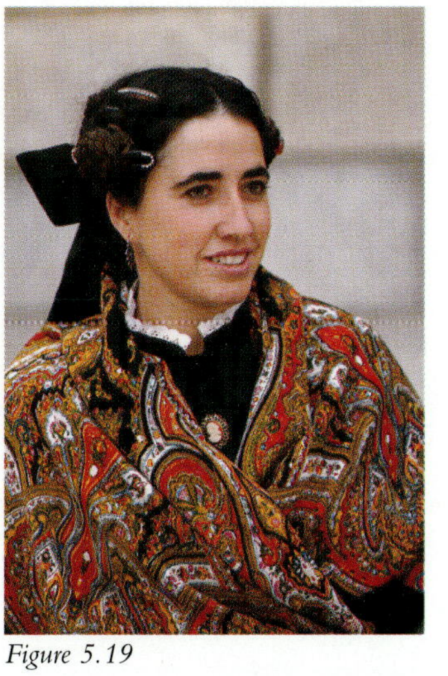

Figure 5.19

Varying facial characteristics

Ethnic characteristics have now become increasingly interbred, particularly in the past 100 years in North America. Facial characteristics that might be accepted in a pure bred ethnic society then become socially undesirable. Films and television have also introduced a Westernized influence which changes social attitudes and fashion.

As surgeons we are now frequently asked to alter or Westernize some ethnic character, and although the wish may be reasonable we must try to appreciate what can be done with harmonious outcome and what would otherwise be unsuited to other facial characters.

Index